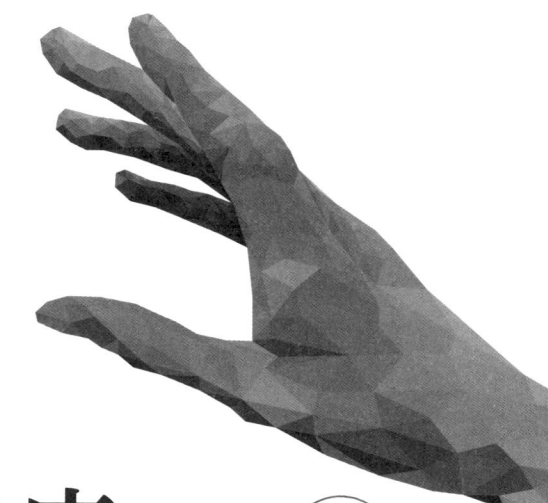

走出巴金森病幽谷
神波刀讓我重拾美好人生

中英對照

Emerging from the Shadows of Parkinson's Disease :
How MRgFUS Restored My Beautiful Life

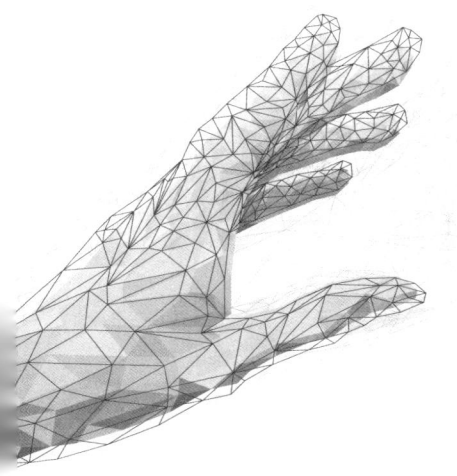

張正駿 —— 著

| 目錄 |

作者序　　　　　　　　　　　　　　　　　3
緣起……　　　　　　　　　　　　　　　　6

壹、發病！
01. 我所罹患的巴金森病　　　　　　　　8
02. 當我發病時……　　　　　　　　　　14

貳、巴金森病的起源與病因？
01. 與巴金森「症」大不相同的病　　　　20
02. 典型的外部運動症狀　　　　　　　　28
03. 引發精神異常與神經障礙　　　　　　32
04. 巴金森病與睡眠障礙　　　　　　　　34

叁、巴金森病的發病中心—大腦
01. 巴金森病的起因　　　　　　　　　　38
02. 巴金森病的診斷　　　　　　　　　　42
03. 巴金森病的藥物治療　　　　　　　　47
04. 腦部深層刺激手術—DBS　　　　　　54

肆、曙光出現—神波刀、聚焦超音波
01. 神波刀的由來與命名　　　　　　　　58
02. 神波刀的治療原理　　　　　　　　　61
03. 神波刀治療顫抖的實例　　　　　　　68
04. 我的神波刀治療經過　　　　　　　　71

伍、治療後……
01. 術後當下的感受　　　　　　　　　　82
02. 一年半過去了……　　　　　　　　　87
03. 感謝　　　　　　　　　　　　　　　90

| 自序 |

破繭而出，重獲新生命

　　我出生在平凡家庭，在體能、智力發展、生活習慣都平衡發揮的狀況下長大，中年之後，也沒有高血壓、血脂、心臟和尿酸等毛病。步入六十歲以後，突然發覺右手會顫抖，隨著時間一年間過一年，顫抖的情況愈來愈明顯，然後右腿部也跟著抖起來。總結這種顫抖的情況，不只是抖動頻率的問題，而是伴隨這手部、腿部肌肉的位移，與無法控制的焦慮。

　　我的祖父、父親和我都是長子，他們也都有顫抖的狀況，父親在九十歲才被診斷為巴金森病，所以我初期認為巴金森病只是造成手會顫抖的病況而已。隨著我自己病況加速進展，加上現代手機查詢功能的提升，我能夠獲取的巴金森病況資訊可以說是非常詳盡，才終於得知我的病情，也知道這種病會繼續惡化，終至癱倒病床，甚至提早死亡，心中的恐懼及焦慮，如巨石壓頂，大到不可復加。

我的恐懼及焦慮來自巴金森病，雖然是老年人易得到的神經性疾病，但它一直是用藥物或復健方式為主的控制，卻不能止住或壓制病情，病患隨著時間會加重病情，所以會形成病患醫療上必須與醫師深刻互動，病患與家人必須付出極大的耐心與體諒。所以這是一個不可逆轉的疾病。我一直覺得擔憂焦躁的是，這個病在現代科技發達的今天，怎麼沒有治癒的良方呢？

我從網路資訊中，得知神波刀的功能，也向醫師詢問，大約過了半年，醫師告訴我可以進行神波刀的醫療。

我事後得知，神波刀可以控制顫抖，但巴金森病患須詳盡的評估，因為巴金森病的發病態樣極為複雜，背後需有醫療團隊加以觀察、分析，提出醫療對策，才能幫助醫師下達精準的診治。剛好我適合神波刀治療，所以在巴金森的眾多病患當中，我算是極為幸運的人。

| 自序 |

/ 自序

　　現在的我，沒有服用藥物，偶而約朋友爬小山，或者一日遊走走逛逛，不再顫抖，肌肉酸痛也消失了，變成原來的我！一般人得了巴金森病，會動作越來越小，越來越少，所以能夠寫下具體描述病況的機率不高；我則是從病後復原的狀態拾筆寫下整個過程，算是對醫療進步的一項回饋。其中真心感謝中國醫藥大學附設醫院整個醫療團隊的耐心付出及精準的醫療，使我得以見證整個巴金森病的全貌，並從中破繭而出，重獲新生命。

　　此書得以出版，是要感謝久陽電腦公司員工們快速的繕打、校正。還要感謝關心我病況的人，我要開心地回應：I Feel So Good！

緣起……

我出生於 1958 年 2 月，於 2025 年出版此書時，我是 67 歲。

2020 年，我在台中市中國醫藥大學附設醫院，首次確定罹患巴金森病（Parkinson's Disease，PD），2022 年 10 月，由中國醫藥大學附設醫院神經科蔡崇豪主任率領的神波刀醫療團隊，為我進行神波刀—聚焦超音波治療。

從步下手術台的這一瞬間，我知道自己罹患的巴金森病，已從我身上完全卸下了！

手術治療後，至今已過了兩年的時間，過往知覺反應從體況逐漸退化，反轉變為快樂過生活；進行神波刀治療之前，普遍認知是巴金森病會讓身體各項機能逐漸走下坡、身體狀況是不可逆轉且無治癒的特效藥。但至今我每日可步行一萬八千多步，在回醫院複診時我更是自豪地向醫師告白：「I Feel Better & Better！（我覺得越來越好）」，我幾乎已經可以正式宣告：「神波刀完全治癒了我的巴金森病！」

壹、發病！

我所罹患的巴金森病

01

在我 30 歲時，我的父親已年屆 60 歲大關。他平日生活極為自律，不菸不酒，不打牌也不應酬，既不吃辣更不喝茶或咖啡，他甚至還會參加中老年人健診，檢測數字除了血壓略低，習慣淺眠，加上偶爾會便祕之外，各項報告數值都非常標準。要求自己早睡早起，每天早晨五點半自行到附近散走，大約七點鐘再返家吃麵包、牛奶當早餐。在我父親所住的公務員社區裡，像他那樣既自律又健康的人，想必是極少數的。但就在我 30 歲時，因為工作穩定，平時有空閒時便關注家人，偶然間發現父親左手會顫抖，比如吃飯時，左手端著碗，右手正要夾菜時，端碗的左手，尤其是靠近指頭，手指拿著碗沿的部位就會上下搖晃，此外就是在陳述某件事情時，雙手若在胸前比劃，便可看到左手手指出現不正常、高頻率的抖動。

根據父親解釋，這是家族遺傳的手抖症，但不會影響健康，因為他除了手抖以外，並未對生活造成任何不良影響。父親65歲退休，常往返台灣與浙江，因為在浙江省還有他的父親，就是我的祖父。家族遺傳手抖之說便是因我父親表示，父執輩從年輕時就會手抖，但卻依舊健康得很，一輩子從未因生病而去看過醫生⋯⋯。

在我印象中，祖父逢人總是笑咪咪的，清瘦且黝黑的體格，習慣把兩個手腕藏在袖子裡，加上飯量很大，有時一餐能吃八顆水煮蛋，而到最後，他是在自然狀態下辭世，享年98歲。

因為父親一直看似健康，加上祖父在世時也一樣，手腳靈活，毫無任何衰退徵兆，故而手抖這件事，很自然地就成為大家生活中的日常。直到2006年，我帶著父親到溪頭風景區去健行，沿途有一些小山坡，大約健行兩個半小時，就在父親吃飯時，我發現他兩手抖動似乎更嚴重，我這時便意識到這個抖動實在不對勁，畢竟在我的眼裡，他這猶如不受控的雙手，到底會不會影響健康？於是，我開始努力尋找各方文獻，極力想為這個毛病下一個註解。

　　然而此時父親仍舊堅持，表示這是家族遺傳的手抖毛病，而且家族成員多半都很長壽，但那時，子女們已然發現箇中關翹，因為醫學文獻裡已經清楚說明，這應該就是巴金森病症。

　　2019 年初，父親在晨間健行中不慎跌倒，住家附近有位史醫師提醒我，老年人跌倒就是一個警訊，絕對不可輕視，建議我應該要帶父親到大型醫院去做個完整的身體檢查。於是，我們選擇到台中榮民總醫院做相關運動神經各科的詳細檢查，神經科當即診斷出父親罹患的就是巴金森病，但因其他各種徵狀皆不明顯，所以並未開立服用藥物，換言之就是醫師認為病況並不算很嚴重。

　　父親當時已經 90 歲，除了雙手顫抖，身體微微前傾，小碎步走路以外,其他並無肉眼可察覺出的異常症狀。而這時我忽然想起,自己似乎也曾出現過幾次手指同時會莫名抖動的狀況,於是當下也請醫生幫我評估一下,醫生叫我做幾個動作,像是蹲下、起身與來回走動、手指運動等,最後結論是並無異常。

2020年春天,父親再度於晨間健行中跌倒,但他跌倒當下,腦子一片空白,不知自己究竟是如何跌倒的?並且對於跌倒之後的事情皆無印象,此後的數天,其體能狀態若用曲線圖來表達,那就是墜崖式的向下曲線,不吃不喝、大小便失禁、眼神無力、整天倒臥床上、拒絕溝通⋯⋯。

我和妹妹先把他送到台中榮總就醫,然後再轉往地區醫院住院並做長期看護,在此期間,他一天服用兩顆醫師開立的處方藥「安滿達」(巴金森病用藥)。但接著卻感染肺炎,所以同時也服用治療肺炎的藥物;除了坐在床頭與人對話之外,其餘時間皆是臥床、睡眠。

最後的幾十天裡,呼吸器及血氧監測都是必要的。

父親在入院五個多月後，於坐臥休息之中自然地離開人世，享壽九十有二歲。

　　在父親的葬禮當中，我手拿麥克風向前來致意的親友們逐一致謝並表達父親一生行誼，之後表弟很好奇地問我，我的雙手為什麼一直在顫抖？我當即毫不猶豫的回答他，我是巴金森病。

　　當時我還未經醫師診斷，但因為情況和父親相同，同時在近幾個禮拜日，我在教堂當司儀時，因為必須手持麥克風，一手要持著儀式程序表作宣達，有時候，右手恍若不受控地抖個不停，唯一的暫停狀態是必須用不抖的左手去按壓顫抖的右手，待壓住幾秒之後，右手才會停止抖動……，而這就是我患病時的初期狀況。

　　此外我也注意到自己的右腳開始出現抖動，右腳在站立時會不由自主地向內縮並往左腳靠攏，然後身體的重心變成在左側，而右腳從大腿延伸到膝蓋，則會出現一些抖動。右手與右腳抖動的差異在於，可以明顯看到右手指尖在顫抖，但右腳反而比較不明顯，兩者較大的差異是大腿部位的抖動時間較短暫。因為我一開始是右手顫抖比較明顯，過了大概半年後，右腳才開始出現上述變化。

當我發病時……

02

當父親過世後不久,我便立志要尋找這個疾病的醫治之道!

我在台灣中部的知名社團擔任幹部,這個社團設立了「健康保健委員會」,延請醫界最知名的醫師與專家定期舉辦「健康講座」,提供企業家們以及他們的家族成員醫療保健上的參考,並且設立**醫療顧問**一職,讓社員們在醫療方面出現疑難雜症時,能有一個窗口可供聯繫諮詢,避免在外面繞了一大圈後,卻仍找不到對應的醫師,徒然延誤病情。

我就是透過醫療顧問林文元醫師的協助,獲得寶貴且正確的診斷與治療。

| 壹. 發病！ |

　　林文元醫師是中國醫藥大學附設醫院的副院長，身兼家庭醫學科的主任，非常瞭解中老年人疾病的態樣，所以在聽完我的陳述後，便轉介我到同屬中國醫藥大學附設醫院神經內科的蔡崇豪主任醫師的門診去就醫。

　　蔡崇豪主任是醫學博士學位，醫學院教授、院長，身兼中國醫藥大學附設醫院神經部巴金森症暨動作障礙科主治醫師，也是國際巴金森症暨動作障礙學會亞太地區執行理事（2017～2021年）。

　　第一次面診大約花了半小時，做雙手畫空圈，食指點鼻子，再點前方的球，腳尖及腳踏地，來回走動的姿態等等，之後再預約時間做腦部斷層攝影等檢查。

　　我當時的不適症狀是右手上臂肌肉向內縮，連睡眠中都會因肌肉痠痛而醒來，空閒時右手手指會顫抖，右腳抖動幅度較輕微，但字卻會愈寫愈小，反倒是走路和講話這兩項功能一如往常，並無任何不適的狀態出現。

　　醫師當時給的處方是：一、確認罹患巴金森病；二、腦部並未受損或器質性病變的狀態；三、暫時先以一天兩次，早晚各服半顆安滿達藥錠來治療；四、巴金森病尚未影響到生活起居。

一開始服用安滿達藥錠，抑制抖動頗見功效，但待三、四個月過後，便開始無法全面壓制症狀，比如抖動現象雖然減輕，顫抖或擺動幅度也變小，但依舊還是會有小幅度的抖動，雙腳也是如此。也就是說，抖動幅度雖會減小，但依然還是會顫抖。

而上手臂的肌肉內縮，依然是我回診的主要訴求症狀，隨後三個月、六個月的回診當中，我竟又發現自己在上大號時，若因雙手過度用力，手部也會顫抖，小便時則因腳部抖動而連帶影響到尿液向左右兩頭噴灑，無法固定尿在同一個點的位置上。我更為此去練氣功，選用一招名為「手抱丹田蹲馬步」的方式來小便，但卻在蹲了幾秒之後，整個身體從右側肩膀開始都到右腳膝蓋，右側身體抖個不停。

還有一次，與家人到清境農場山區遊玩，大家因為沒有弄清楚路線，所以越走越遠，我當下與家人意見相左,又急著想趕快走出迷路的困境,一時緊張,身體右側又開始抖個不停,而且顫抖幅度非常大,甚至把自己都嚇了一跳;還有一次參與小型登山,帶著登山杖,若右手持杖,因為手抖就換到左手持杖,如此左右手交換了好幾回,還是有眼尖隊友發現,直言告訴我這是巴金森病症,當下被說得有點覺得自尊心受損。最糟糕的情況是,難免有開車載朋友的時候,但擺在方向盤上的右手不自覺的抖動起來,對方就會問:「你的手怎麼啦?」

我從網路查詢中得知,「神波刀」在台灣被用來治療巴金森病與顫抖症,遂向蔡崇豪主任提出這種治療的請求,蔡主任向我說明了神波刀治療的方向,但建議我再觀察自身病況一段時間後再說。

就在2022年的5月～8月之間,我的巴金森病迅速惡化,一天服用兩顆的安滿達藥錠已擋不住顫抖狀況,抖動變得無時不在,自己也開始出現情緒低落,不愛說話,聲調變得更加低沉,吃東西容易嗆到,就連騎腳踏車時,右邊腳掌不會順著踩踏的慣性,很容易脫出腳踏板。手的持重力也逐漸減弱，當右手拿著馬克杯時，右手抖動會造成杯內的水溢出來，林林總總的狀況，真是讓我感覺相當的苦惱。

我從醫學文獻中得知，巴金森病會一路惡化、僵直、癱倒病床、直至死亡，心中恐懼的陰影愈加沉重，揮之不去。除了巴金森病之外，我的身體狀況一直保持很好，血壓始終維持在 75～120 mm Hg（毫米汞柱），心跳率則是在 70～80 之間，加上身高 174cm，體重 75Kg，並無三高問題，也無尿酸過高的疑慮，大小便與睡眠狀態一直都維持正常，沒有抽菸，沒有飲酒，一天一杯咖啡，偶而與朋友登登小山。

2021 年做過全身正子攝影檢查，除了發現頸部甲狀腺有小粒結節，後經過超音波及穿刺檢查，確定是良性，此外便沒有再發現身體有任何不良的狀況。

這大概要歸功於我的樂天性格，凡事樂觀看待，但巴金森病卻讓我真實承受了巨大的生死壓力！！

貳、巴金森病的起源與病因？

與巴金森「症」大不相同的病 01

　　巴金森症是一個較廣泛性的專業術語，描述了一組動作障礙症狀（動作遲緩、震顫、肌肉僵硬、姿勢不穩）。這些症狀可能由各種情況引起，包括巴金森病、其它神經退化性疾病、藥物或毒素。所謂的巴金森病是一種漸進性的神經退化性疾病，其病理機制是腦幹中產生多巴胺的神經元大量喪失，導致產生動作遲緩、僵硬、顫抖等症狀。

　　巴金森病與老人失智症和中風三者，並列為老人三大疾病，其主要特徵是：

1. 待達到一定年齡後，便很容易出現。
2. 有一定程度的高比例。

貳、巴金森病的起源與病因？

3. 男女都有可能患病且很難治癒，更會影響生活。

神經系統疾病是失能的主要原因，而阿茲海默症（失智症）和巴金森病是老年人中最常見的兩種神經系統退化性疾病。巴金森病的特徵是動作障礙，包括無法控制的靜止性震顫，肢體僵硬，平衡感不佳和運動功能衰退等。此外，還有種類繁多的非運動症狀，造成生活上的困擾，有些甚至早在動作症狀發生之前就出現了，例如便祕、憂鬱、嗅覺消失、習慣在睡夢中舞動手腳等。在台灣，此病好發的年紀平均約 60～62 歲，此一族群盛行率約 1%，男性發病機率為女性的 1.5 倍，推估目前在台灣 2,300 萬人口中，約有 3～5 萬名左右的病人。

巴金森病的主要病理變化是，中腦的黑質組織多巴胺神經元退化死亡，動作障礙的原因是腦內多巴胺分泌不足，如果將人體大腦運動區比喻為全身的動作指揮中心，基底核（在本書第叁章中另有詳述）就如同參謀總長辦公室，而多巴胺就像傳令兵的基地；巴金森病患者的指揮系統，因為培訓基地無法培育足夠的傳令兵，導致訊息傳遞紊亂，送出的指令不足，讓指揮中心無法正常的帶領肢體完成日常動作[1]。

此病症最早是由英國醫師詹姆斯・巴金森（James Parkinson）發現並記錄。巴金森病是一種漸進式惡化的疾病，會逐步影響病人的神經系統以及由神經支配的各種部位。巴金森病好發於中老年人，但也有青壯年罹病的案例。50歲以前發病的病人稱為年輕型巴金森病，年輕型的病程較慢，癒後狀況也比較好（部分內容取材自網路搜尋：帕金森氏症自我檢測與常見五大疑問）。

根據「維基百科」的說明，巴金森病是一種影響中樞神經系統的慢性神經退化疾病，主要影響運動神經功能，症狀通常隨時間緩慢出現，早期最明顯的症狀為顫抖、肢體僵硬、運動功能減退和步態異常，也可能有認知和行為問題；至於失智症在病情嚴重的巴金森患者中相當常見，超過 1 ／ 3 的病例也會發生重度抑鬱障礙和焦慮症，可能會伴隨包括知覺、睡眠、情緒問題等症狀。

巴金森病的成因截至目前還不清楚，但普遍認為和

貳、巴金森病的起源與病因？

遺傳與環境因子相關。家族中曾有罹患巴金森病病史的人，通常較可能得到此病，此外暴露於特定農藥、曾有頭部外傷者者，患病風險也比較高；反觀有吸菸習慣、常喝咖啡或飲茶者，患病風險則相對較低。巴金森病主要的運動症狀導因於中腦黑質細胞死亡，使患者相關腦區的多巴胺不足。細胞死亡的原因目前瞭解甚少，但已知和神經元蛋白質組成路易氏體的過程有關。典型的巴金森病主要靠症狀診斷，神經成像也能協助排除其他疾病的可能性。

　　巴金森症是一種運動型症候群，為數種症狀類似的運動障礙合稱。定義上，症狀必須有運動遲緩（例如自主性運動減退，或重複性動作的速率及靈活度下降，像是自發性手指輕敲），再加入一項上述的下列症狀：鉛筆樣僵直（Lead-Pipe）、齒輪樣僵直（Cogwheel）（意指當你在病人放鬆情況下，扳動他的手腳，仍會感到像咯咯般齒輪一樣的阻力）、靜態顫抖及姿勢不穩等，可根據以上成因，區分為以下四種型態：

一、原發性

二、次級或後天獲得

三、遺傳性

四、巴金森附加症候群（例如多重系統退化症、皮質基底核退化症）

巴金森病則是指原發性的巴金森症，意即沒有明確可辨別的成因，同時也是最常見的一種病症。近年來發現數個基因與巴金森病有直接關聯，這與原先以原發性疾病為準的定義產生衝突，因此，一般也將和巴金森病程類似的遺傳性巴金森症納入其中，並用「家族巴金森病」和「偶發性巴金森病」來區別遺傳性和真正病因不明的病人族群。

「巴金森病」通常歸類為運動性疾病，但它也會引起其他非運動性的症狀，例如感覺障礙、認知困難和睡眠障礙。「巴金森附加症候群」則是在巴金森病狀的基礎外還有其他附加臨床徵候，這類疾病主要包括多重系統退化、進行性上眼神經核麻痺、大腦皮質基底退化和路易氏體失智症等。

「路易體失智症」是一種與巴金森病類似的突觸核蛋白病變，包括出現幻覺、注意力起伏不定、行動遲緩、步伐不穩、或運動功能減退。其失智症狀可出現於巴金森症狀已現或之後的頭一年。此病症和巴金森病合併失智症非常類似，然而這兩種疾病的關係目前仍有待進一步研究釐清。它們可被視為兩種不同的疾病，也能被視為一種疾病卻在不同面向上的展現。

由此看來，我所罹患的巴金森病，透過遺傳所導致的可能性居多。

2015 年，全球約有 620 萬人患有巴金森病，並且造成 11.7 萬人死亡。巴金森病通常發生在 60 歲以上的老人，約有 1% 的老人罹患該病；男性較女性容易得到巴金森病。若患者在小於 50 歲發病，則稱為早發性巴金森病。巴金森病造成患者健康威脅的風險因子包括認知功能減退和失智、吞嚥障礙、老年發病和較嚴重的疾病狀態。另一方面，以顫抖為主要症狀的患者，較肢體僵硬為主的患者有更高的存活率。巴金森病患者因吸入性肺炎導致死亡的機率，大約是一般人的兩倍。此病以英國醫生詹姆斯・巴金森為名，他在 1817 年發表了《論震顫性麻痺》（An Essay on the Shaking Palsy）一書，書中首次詳述了六個巴金森病的相關症狀，他的生日 4 月 11 日也因此定為世界巴金森日，社群團體會在當天舉行公眾推廣活動，而鬱金香則是巴金森病的象徵符號。一些著名患者的病情提高了大眾對此病的關注，包括中華人民共和國領導人鄧小平、演員麥可・J・福克斯、奧林匹克自行車手戴維斯・菲尼和職業拳擊手穆罕莫德・阿里（本章節部分內容取材自網路搜尋：維基百科／帕金森氏症／分類）。

　　但是巴金森病很容易讓人聯想到阿茲海默失智症，這兩種症狀不同，但因屬老年疾病，有人在老年時同時罹患這兩種症狀。巴金森病與阿茲海默症同屬中樞神經退化性疾病。兩者的差異在於阿茲海默症是大腦海馬迴和大腦皮層的神經細胞退化，導致認知功能障礙。而巴金森病則是中腦黑質的神經細胞退化，症狀主要是以行動和肢體障礙的方式表現，兩者的病症差異可見下表所示[2]。

	巴金森病	阿茲海默症
病因	中腦黑質的神經細胞退化所致。	大腦海馬迴和大腦皮層的神經細胞退化所致。
症狀表現	肢體症狀為主，包括手抖、肌肉僵硬、動作遲緩以及姿態異常等。	認知障礙為主，症狀包括記憶力變差、說話表達能力異常、喪失時間觀念、判斷力變差、情緒起伏大、個性改變以及活動力變差等。
發病年紀	大多在50歲以上，少部分在45歲以下。	大多在65歲以上發病，極少數因為基因變異會在30～60歲間發病。
治療方法	藥物治療為主，也可用手術治療改善症狀。	藥物治療為主，多使用能改善知能的藥物，如愛憶欣、憶思能等。

製表：作者
資料來源：轉載自〈帕金森氏症剛開始6前兆、症狀檢測、治療、壽命，一次看〉網路文章。

典型的外部運動症狀 02

　　巴金森病有四種主要運動症狀：顫抖、肢體僵硬、動作遲緩、姿勢不穩。

　　顫抖是最明顯且最為人所知的症狀，約有 30% 的巴金森病患在剛患病時不會出現顫抖，但隨著病程進展，多數患者會逐漸產生此症狀。巴金森病的顫抖通常是靜止性顫抖，也就是四肢在靜止狀態時的抖動最明顯，但睡覺或有意識移動四肢時，症狀反而會消失。

　　顫抖對四肢遠端的影響較大，剛發病時通常只有一隻手或一隻腳出現症狀，但隨後會擴及雙手及雙腳。巴金森病的顫抖經常伴隨有「搓藥丸」的手部動作，也就是患者食指會不自主向大拇指靠攏，使兩指互相繞圈圈，就好像藥師在做藥丸一般。

運動功能減退症是巴金森病的另一種特徵，患者動作變慢，且會影響從運動起始到執行的整個過程。患者無法做出連續動作或同步執行不同的動作。而運動遲緩症（Bradykinesia）則屬於運動功能減退症的一種，強調運動執行過程的動作緩慢，是巴金森病早期最常見的症狀。患者最初會在執行日常生活的精細動作（如寫字、縫紉或梳妝）時遇到困難；臨床評估則多半會要求患者做出類似上述的動作來觀察。運動遲緩症造成的影響，隨動作種類和患者身心狀態而異，影響程度受到患者活動力和情緒狀態的影響，導致有些患者嚴重到無法走路，但有些患者卻還能騎自行車。一般而言，巴金森病患者在治療後，多半都能改善運動遲緩的症狀。

肢體的僵硬是由於患者肌張力增加，肌肉持續收縮，導致四肢移動困難。巴金森病造成的肢體僵硬，可能是鉛筆管型僵硬（阻力固定）或齒輪型僵硬（阻力不固定但具規則性）齒輪型僵硬，則可能是顫抖結合肌張力增加造成的。巴金森病早期患者的肢體僵硬常是不對稱的，並且好發於頸部和肩膀，隨著擴及顏面和四肢，最後隨病程進展蔓延到全身，使患者逐漸失去運動能力。我感覺到我的運動狀態和此有關，尤其是騎自行車時，右腳經常會掉出踏板以外，無法順順地踩踏自行車。

姿態不穩是巴金森病晚期的症狀之一，患者可能因平衡感不佳而經常跌倒，並可能因此骨折。疾病初期通常不會有姿態不穩的現象。高達40%的患者於病程中曾因姿態不穩跌倒，跌倒的次數則與病情嚴重程度有關。我個人的患病過程中因為步行還算正常，所以並未發生過跌倒的狀況。

不寧腿症後群（RLS）是一種常見的運動障礙，主要指小腿深部休息時，小腿出現無法忍受的不適，包括小腿劇烈疼痛、異常感覺等。不寧腿症後群（RLS）在巴金森病患者中常見，其發病率可達8%～34%，它通過干擾睡眠和睡眠維持來影響患者的睡眠品質。其發病機制可能與多巴胺能系統障礙、基因變異、鐵代謝異常等方面相關。

　　此外,其他動作障礙症狀包括姿態、說話與吞嚥異常。患者為避免跌倒可能產生慌張步態(例如走路時加速步伐且姿態前屈),也可能出現發聲困難、面具臉(撲克臉)或字越寫越小,導致患者可能以此產生各種運動問題(本章節部分內容參考及抄錄自網路搜尋:維基百科／帕金森氏症／運動症狀)。

引發精神異常與神經障礙 03

　　少數巴金森病患者可能產生輕度到重度的神經性精神疾患，包括言語、認知、情緒、行為和思考混亂。

　　疾病中後期可能有認知混亂的現象，且發生比率隨得病時間增加。巴金森病患者較常見的認知缺陷問題為執行困難，這將使患者在計畫、認知彈性、抽象思考、規則理解、做出適當行為、工作記憶、專注力等方面都受到影響；其他認知困難症狀還包括注意力渙散、時間感受和估計不準確、認知處理緩慢等問題。患者的記憶力會受到影響，尤其難以回憶先前學習的訊息；然而，若提供線索輔助患者回憶，則能改善相關的症狀。失去空間感是另一種可能的症狀，檢驗中會要求患者辨識臉

| 貳、巴金森病的起源與病因？ |

部表情和畫線的方向，藉此判斷患者是否有此類障礙。

　　巴金森病患者罹患失智症的風險，約為一般人的二至六倍，且發生率隨患病時間增加。失智症導致患者和照顧者的生活品質降低，並讓病患死亡率增高，通常更需住進療養院。

　　相較於一般人，沒有認知障礙的巴金森病患者較容易有行為和情緒障礙，且這些患者通常沒有失智症。最常見的情緒障礙有憂鬱症、冷漠和焦慮。然而，巴金森病患者常會有失智症、臉部表情減少、運動功能減退、冷漠和發生困難等症狀，這使得要診斷出情緒障礙變得更加複雜。我回憶自己在患病過程中，也有對於複雜的事情缺乏耐心，也會習慣推脫，不願意去面對的情況（本章節部分內容參考及抄錄自網路搜尋：維基百科／帕金森氏症／神經性精神病患）。

巴金森病與睡眠障礙

04

睡眠障礙也是巴金森病患者可能出現的一種病徵，治療用的藥物可能會惡化相關問題。患者會有嗜睡、快速動眼期中斷、失眠等現象，「維基百科」敘述一份系統性回顧報告顯示13%的巴金森病患者有睡眠障礙問題。

日間過度嗜睡（ESD）是指，患者日間清醒時竟沒有預兆地又突然入睡。目前，ESD發病機制尚未明確，可能與上行網狀系統功能障礙有關。據研究報導，約有50%巴金森病患者受ESD的影響，男性、生性抑鬱者更屬常見。在某些情況下，ESD對患者日常生活的影響，甚至比巴金森病的運動症狀還要大。

快速動眼睡眠期行為障礙（RBD）是一種與快動眼

睡眠（REM）相關的異常睡眠行為。這是一種以夢境相關為特徵的睡眠模式，RBD 患者睡眠中通常伴隨恐懼和暴力，同時在 REM 期，可能會出現快速肌肉抽搐及肢體亂動揮舞的現象。

我的巴金森病狀倒是在睡眠問題上並無多大關聯。記得我在工作時幾乎沒有睡午覺的習慣，但在夜間睡眠休息時則是很好入睡，也極少做惡夢。通常會打斷睡眠的，主要是右上臂肌肉的內縮和右腳的肌肉想要伸展。

多數巴金森病患者病因不明，只有小部分可歸因於遺傳因子。專家普遍比較認可的說法是，巴金森病發病不是單因子引起，而是多種因子共同參與，包括環境因子、年齡因子、遺傳因子等，其他風險因子也可能和巴金森病有關，但其因果關係尚未被證實（本章節部分內容參考及抄錄自網路搜尋：維基百科／帕金森氏症／睡眠障礙）。

---

1. 馬偕紀念醫院老人醫學團隊，神經科資深主治醫師陳培豪撰〈認識巴金森病的診斷與治療〉，馬偕院訊—2020 年 6 月第 367 期，P16-17。
2. 轉載自〈帕金森氏症剛開始 6 前兆、症狀檢測、治療、壽命，一次看〉網路文章。

叁、巴金森病的發病中心—大腦

巴金森病的起因

01

　　常見的巴金森病症狀，比如顫抖、身體僵硬、動作遲緩、平衡障礙、臉部表情僵硬沒有笑容，比較有憂鬱症現象，這些都跟大腦基底核有關，基底核是大腦訊號的轉運中樞。歸根究底，大腦的損傷一開始都是從自由基而來，自由基會影響粒腺體，粒腺體是細胞產生能量的地方，所謂的細胞發電廠被自由基干擾以後，產生的能量就變差，容易退化。

　　大腦中有一個地方叫黑質（是中腦的一個神經核團），黑質中有一個部位叫緻密部，是分泌多巴胺的地方，此處很容易受到路易小體的傷害，受到迫害後就無法分泌多巴胺，順勢直接影響我們的基底核，產生功能上的障礙，畢竟大腦許多執行功能都須要經過基底核，就好比一個董事長和總經理的角色，董事長的經營理念要透過總經理去執行，待評估 OK 後放行，類似開紅燈或綠燈的角色，分泌足夠的多巴胺就開綠燈，簡而言之就是走直路；另一個間接路徑是踩剎車的角色，或直接說就是給紅燈。缺乏多巴胺的病人沒有辦法開綠燈，這時想要走路，邁出的第一步往往會停頓很久、會延遲，所以踏出去的時候會比較慢，邁出去第一步以後就會開始一直跟著走，不只在動作、思考上，就算是在認知功能上也會變得比較慢，因為我們大腦的思考也會經過基底核[1]。

　　巴金森病的主要症狀大多肇因於黑質緻密部的多巴胺性神經元退化。大腦基底核與外界聯繫的路徑大致依其投射位置可分為五條，分別為動作迴路、動眼迴路、聯合皮質迴路、邊緣系統迴路和眼眶額葉皮質迴路。由於巴金森病會影響基底核上游訊息的傳遞，因此前述的所有迴路都可能會受到波及，使得巴金森病患者會出現動作、注意力和學習上的障礙（上述部分內容參考及截錄自網路搜尋：維基百科／帕金森氏症／病理生理學）。

　　1980 年，運動迴路的理論雛形問世，該迴路與巴金森病的關聯性被提出，這對當時的科學界帶來極大影響。雖然事後發現該模型無法解釋某些現象，因此做了一些修正。在這個模型中，基底核負責調控運動系統，以避免其於不適當的時機活化。當大腦確定要做某個動作時，基底核會減少抑制信號，使動作能順利執行。而多巴胺可以抑制來自基底核的抑制訊息，因此多巴胺濃度高時，能促使運動指令順利發生，多巴胺濃度低時，運動指令就會受到基底核的抑制。

　　巴金森病患者的中樞神經多巴胺濃度較低，因而造成運動功能減退。基於此項理論，藥物治療上常會選用提升多巴胺濃度的藥品，但這樣的結果也常導致運動系統在不恰當的時機點被活化，造成身體不自主的運動（以上部分內容參考及截錄自網路搜尋：維基百科／帕金森氏症／病理生理學）。

從病理上來說，巴金森病患者「中腦的黑質神經細胞」退化，以致無法分泌神經傳導物質「多巴胺」，而由於缺乏多巴胺，人體才會無法有效傳達大腦下達的指令。

巴金森病的診斷

　　許多名人得到巴金森病,例如教宗保祿二世、葛理翰牧師、美國前司法部長李諾、葛萊美獎紅星琳達‧朗斯黛、世界拳王阿里、好萊塢明星麥可‧J‧福克斯（Michael J. Fox）、曾獲奧林匹克運動會自行銅牌的戴維斯‧菲尼、羅賓‧威廉斯、鄧小平、希特勒、台灣音樂人李泰祥、女星方岑、歌手詹雅雯、抗議名人柯賜海等。

　　巴金森病是一種漸進式惡化的疾病,會逐步影響病人的神經系統,以及由神經支配的各個部位。巴金森病好發於中老年人,但也有青壯年罹病的案例。

　　巴金森病其實有跡可循,如果能盡早發現並接受治療，效過往往也較好。台灣動作障礙學會提供簡單的「巴金森病自我檢測表」，讓民眾可在家自我檢驗，如果以下十種情況中若有出現三個，那便有可能是罹患初期巴金森病的前兆，建議找神經內科醫師諮詢。

一、你的雙手是否曾經在休息放鬆時，出現顫抖的情形？

二、走路時有一隻手臂彎曲且不會擺動？

三、身體在站立或行進時，姿勢會向前彎曲？

四、走路姿勢雜亂、不順，好像打結了或一腳拖在後面？

五、寫字變慢而且字體變小？

六、步伐小且常常跌倒？

七、常覺得懶洋洋，做甚麼事情都沒有動力？

八、頸部後方或是肩膀常常疼痛？

九、刻意地避免與聊不來的朋友或家人相處？

十、音調出現變化？變得更單調、小聲或沙啞？

巴金森病的症狀因人而異，惡化速度亦差異甚大，巴金森病會出現的症狀包括：

一、手抖、肢體顫抖：除了肢體顫抖外，病人還可能出現摩擦手指的動作。

二、肌肉僵硬：病人全身肌肉都可能出現僵硬的狀況，會使病人的活動變得困難。

三、行動遲緩：病人的動作變得緩慢，以前很簡單的動作現在要更費時費力才能完成。走路的步伐縮小，甚至有時會用小碎步或拖著腿的方式走路。

四、平衡感變差：因為肌肉僵硬和顫抖連帶使病人平衡感不佳，增加跌倒受傷的風險。

五、言語變化：說話聲音改變、講話含糊不清或說話前猶豫不決。

六、難以做精細的動作：一些精細的動作會受到影響，例如做菜、寫字或彈奏樂器等。

巴金森病可依照病人運動失調的嚴重度分為五期，以下介紹不同期別的差異。

第一期：病人的單側肢體出現症狀，但對生活無礙。

第二期：病人的雙側肢體雖然出現症狀，但還能維持平衡。

第三期：病人難以維持穩定的姿勢，容易跌倒。

第四期：病人只能勉強站立，日常生活開始需要有他人照護。

第五期（末期）：病人需長期臥床或用輪椅代步，日常生活需要專業照服人員照顧 [2]。

巴金森病雖然是常見的疾病，但在疾病非常早期的階段，或是在年紀較大的病人身上，診斷往往較為困難，醫師通常要進行詳細的疾病問診病史及神經學檢查之後，才會做出診斷判決。

某一些疾病的症狀亦類似巴金森病，患者走路遲緩、僵直或顫抖，包括腦中風、水腦症、腦部腫瘤、失智症、抗精神病藥物副作用、病毒性腦炎、腦外傷、甲狀腺功能低下、維他命 B12 缺乏等，須與巴金森病作鑑別診斷 [3]。

有充足的臨床證據指出，若是常常跌倒、症狀進展迅速、對於抗巴金森藥物沒有反應等，都較可能是類巴金森症候群，而非巴金森病。因此必須藉由醫師安排相關的抽血檢驗及腦部影像檢查，如電腦斷層（CT）、核磁共振攝影（MRI）或腦部多巴胺神經元斷層造影（TRODAT）等，來做相關的鑑別診斷[3]。

叁、巴金森病的發病中心—大腦

巴金森病的藥物治療

03

　　巴金森病是種退化性疾病，出現僵硬、顫抖、動作變慢、平衡困難等症狀，代表腦部已經退化到一定程度，就要接受治療，及早接受治療有助延緩疾病進展。若發現手抖，除了巴金森病外，還可能是神經病變、腦部腫瘤或甲狀腺問題等。確定診斷巴金森病後，便要積極接受治療。

　　腦中的多巴胺不只調控動作，還可調控情緒、睡眠等。因此除了大家較熟悉的動作症狀外，巴金森病還可能出現許多非動作症狀，例如情緒低落、便秘、疼痛、睡眠障礙、嗅覺改變等，有些非動作症狀會比動作症狀更早出現，若發現有相關，也要就醫檢查。

巴金森病是個慢性病，隨著病情進展，藥物需要適時調整，因此就近就醫是確保能規律回診與醫師討論的關鍵之一。接受巴金森病治療後，病人、家屬可以記錄用藥日記，包括用藥時間、動作症狀、非動作症狀、睡眠狀況、可能的副作用等。在回診時，醫師便能根據用藥日記，評估是否需要調整藥物 4。

　　巴金森病在之前是無法治癒的，初期症狀常用左多巴藥物（Levodopa）治療，當左多巴效果降低後則配合使用多巴胺激動劑。隨著病程惡化，神經元將持續流失，因此必須隨之增加藥物劑量，但藥量剛增加時又會產生以不自主的異動症副作用（本節主要參考及抄錄自網路搜尋：維基百科／帕金森氏症／治療）。

　　用藥時的劑量波動會對患著生活造成嚴重影響。患者剛用藥時，體內劑量較高，因此患者的症狀較和緩，此時稱為「通電狀態」（亦即「On」State）；反之，在藥效降低後患者的運動性症狀又會出現，此時稱為「斷電狀態」（亦即「Off」State）。過高劑量的左多巴會使患者產生異動症，無限制提高藥物劑量並非將藥物濃度控制於「通電狀態」的方法 。因此須以其他方法延長藥物在體內滯留的時間，方法包含合併使用多巴胺受體促效劑及 MAO-B 受體抑制劑，以往醫師會藉由暫時停用左多巴以減少運動性症狀，但該作法可能導致巴金森高熱症候群之致命性的副作用，所以現在已不再使用。目前有廠商發展出靜脈內及腸道內的緩釋技術，讓左多巴能穩定且緩慢地釋放。研究顯示，緩釋劑比起傳統劑型能有效減少異動症的情形，多數患者終身必須服用左多巴，但服用劑量較大的患者，日後有可能會遇到本品的運動性副作用（本節主要參考及抄錄自網路搜尋：維基百科／帕金森氏症／治療）。

目前，巴金森病的治療方式有藥物治療、外科手術、聚焦超音波治療、物理治療、語言治療等。其中，藥物治療主要是回復多巴胺的活性，使基底核能保持正常運作。目前治療的藥物共有六大類，包含了左多巴（Levodopa）、多巴胺受體促效劑、單胺氧化酵素抑制劑、

N-甲基-D-天門冬胺酸受體 NMDA 促效劑、兒茶酚-O-甲基轉移、COMT 抑制劑及抗乙醯膽鹼激素，而左多巴是目前最有效也歷史最悠久的藥物之一。[3]

臨床醫師考量患者的症狀，只要做適度的藥物搭配，初期都可以達到所謂「蜜月期」的效果，有些患者甚至可以達到看不太出有病症的情形。

左多巴（Levodopa）是巴金森病的主要治療藥物，已被開發且廣泛使用近 60 年。左多巴會由體內的多巴胺脫羧 （Dopa Decarboxylase）代謝爲多巴胺（Dopamine）在腸胃道會產生噁心、嘔吐等副作用，在關節組織則會產生僵硬等副作用，最後只有不到 10% 的左多巴能夠到達腦部並發揮療效。當年爲了提高左多巴到達腦部的濃度，羅氏藥廠取得 Benserazide 的專利，默克藥廠取得 Carbidopa 的專利，兩者皆爲抑制周邊組織中多巴胺脫羧酶的活性，並與左多巴混製成口服劑型（商品名分別爲：美道普錠 Madopar、心寧美錠 Sinemet），藉以提高腦部左多巴的濃度，同時減少巴金森病的藥丸負擔。

| 叁、巴金森病的發病中心—大腦 |

　　恩他卡朋（諾康停膜衣錠）Entacapone 為一種 COMT 抑制劑，主要作用是抑制兒茶酚 -O- 甲基轉移酶（Catechol-O-Methyl Transferase）也是在體內代謝左多巴而導致左多巴無法到達腦部的另一種酵素。2003 年美國上市的始立膜衣錠 stavelo，進一步將 Entacapone 與左多巴胺及瑞多寧緩釋膠囊 carbidopa 混製成口服劑型，進一步減少巴金森氏病的藥丸負擔。其主要臨床試驗 First Step（2005 年～ 2007 年）為多國多中心（包含歐盟及美國）的雙盲隨機臨床試驗，結果顯示對於改善症狀的效果優於左多巴及 Carbidopa 混製口服劑型。

　　雖然長期抑制多巴胺脫羧　並未發現嚴重的不良反應，目前仍是主要的治療藥物，但抑制兒茶酚 -O- 甲基轉移的藥物，可就沒有那麼幸運了。一種抑制兒茶酚 -O- 甲基轉移的藥物托卡朋 Tolcapone，已因可能導致肝毒性而下市，而 Entacapone 也可能會提高肝功能不良，或讓酗酒病人的肝指數達兩倍以上。

　　抑制全身的某種酵素來達成特定藥物到特定目標器

官的藥劑設計,容易衍生不必要的全身性副作用,就好比從家裡到某地,因為怕路上被狗咬,所以不考慮搭車前往,卻將所有流浪狗都捉起來,但如果流浪狗可以趕小偷,那麼若將流浪狗通通關起來,那麼小偷豈不就變多了。因此,最近藥物開發已朝向藥物載體的概念努力,將治療藥物載入特定載體,就像是坐車到目的地一樣,為了避免被流浪狗攻擊,還可加裝隱形或防彈等系統。

為了減少巴金森病的藥丸負擔,經皮膚吸收的藥物也陸續被開發。透過皮膚將藥物送入體內,角質層是最大的障礙,傳統方式是破壞或軟化角質層,如辣椒膏即是由破壞角質層來提高藥物輸送,近來藥物載體的概念逐漸被導入,奈米化載體可使特定藥物停留在特定皮層中持續緩慢輸出,甚至可達數十天之久。

目前已上市,經皮吸收多巴胺致效劑貼片（Transdermal Dopaminergic patches）,為在美國上市的紐普洛寧皮貼片劑 Transdermal Patch Neupro®。在歐盟上市的卡比多巴和左旋多巴的複方藥 Duodopa,臨床試驗顯示 Duodopa 由小腸緩慢吸收。此二者可有效降低異動症（Dyskinesia）或突然斷電（Off Phenomenon）所導致的身體僵直，並可改善續電時間（On Phenomenon）及降低波動現象（On-Off Fluctuation）。有關巴金森病的治療，可參閱台灣動作障礙學會的巴金森病治療建議 [5]。

　　藥丸負擔不只是巴金森病患才有，許多慢性病用藥都有這個問題。透過藥物輸送系統的研究開發，減少藥丸顆數及降低全身性副作用，並非夢想，相信不久的將來，全面個人化藥物治療的新時代即將來臨，任何慢性病只要戴個手錶，插入個人疾病卡就可得到持續的藥物輸送治療，病人不必再承擔服用過多藥丸所造成的副作用 [6]。

腦部深層刺激手術—DBS

這種手術將一個神經刺激器置入腦中,刺激器再以電衝動刺激特定腦區。一般會推薦運動症狀時好時壞而呈現反覆波動的病人接受腦深層刺激手術,對於藥物控制不佳或無法接受藥物的顫抖病人也很適合(本節主要參考及抄錄自網路搜尋:維基百科/帕金森氏症/手術)。

第一線都是以藥物治療原發性顫抖及巴金森病靜止性顫抖,但當部分病患藥物控制的效果不好或是引發嚴重的藥物副作用時,就會考慮用深腦刺激手術(Deep Brain Stimulation Surgery,DBS)來治療。

此術是需進手術房做立體定位手術以及局部麻醉,

由開顱手術植入一個細長的電極導線到腦的特定神經核，例如視丘下核，以電刺激調節大腦迴路的運作，改善運動功能；同時要在胸前皮下埋入電池，以供應腦內電極所需電流，因此約三至四年，需重新換電池，由於需要開腦植入電線、電極、裝皮下電池，許多病人心存害怕或是對電線過敏或是擔心開腦的副作用而裹足不前（台大校訊第 1542 期／顫抖不再～台大醫院認識「神波刀」記者會）。

　　第一次手術治療需要部分自費，但台灣健保署提供終生電池更換給付，手術風險低、併發症少。但須注意深腦刺激手術並不是治癒疾病的手術，而是需要隨著時間與症狀需求來調整刺激模組，並搭配藥物來達到進一步治療效果 7。

　　我在收到磁振導航聚焦超音波（MRgFUS）之前的資料中，發現腦深層刺激術是選項之一，但因這個手術更加複雜且不是一勞永逸，恐造成病患心中更大的陰影，故而終究沒有採用。

| 走出巴金森病幽谷:神波刀讓我重拾美好人生 |

1. 李政家 Karl Li ,DC,PT 「作伙來開講」:粒腺體與巴金森病。
2. 轉載自〈帕金森氏症剛開始6前兆、症狀檢測、治療、壽命,一次看〉網路文章。
3. 馬偕紀念醫院老人醫學團隊,神經科資深主治醫師陳培豪撰〈認識巴金森氏症的診斷與治療〉,馬偕院訊—2020年6月第367期,P16-17。
4. 上述部分內容參考天下雜誌文-照護線上,天下部落格,2024年1月11日。「輕微手抖就要治療,避免快速惡化~每月自我檢測提早發現帕金森氏症」。
5. 台灣動作障礙學會巴金森病治療建議,Ac Ta Neuroloica Taiwanica,2023;32:145-184(台灣神經學雜誌)
6. 轉載自中國醫藥大學附設醫院蔡銘駿醫師撰〈不想再當藥罐子!巴金森病藥物治療新發展〉,《中國醫訊》第130期。
7. 台大醫院巴金森病醫療中心簡介「神波刀~聚焦超音波!!」

肆、曙光出現──神波刀、聚焦超音波

神波刀的由來與命名 01

2022 年 8 月的例行回診，蔡崇豪醫師告訴我，我可以進行神波刀治療。

這對我來說真是一個好消息，我從被觀察名單晉級到核可名單中，也等於從急劇惡化的巴金森病裡，由瀕臨死亡幽谷變成看見一道曙光。為什麼它在我的認知上是這麼地有份量呢？從既有的文獻上記載：

一、它是利用非侵入性的聚焦超音波束，在病灶處進行腦內的熱消融。

二、不需要全身或半身麻醉。

三、對於顫抖性為主的巴金森病，可以改善。以目前的文獻資料顯示，治療過後的四年內，療效維持不墜[1]。

更何況在此之前，是沒有可以逆轉此病的對策。

雖然醫師說這是新式的治療，不知有無復發的風險，但我深知這種教學大型醫療機構，有台灣衛生主管機關核定的醫療行為，再加上數十年來巴金森病從不可逆轉的下墜式病情，走到終於見到有逆轉之機，我當然馬上就答應參與治療。

臺灣已步上高齡化社會的趨勢，原發性顫抖及巴金森病患人數逐年增加。整體而言，光是原發性顫抖症的盛行率，在每一百萬人中約有四千至四萬人的罹病人口；而在 60 歲以上的老年人口中，其盛行率更高達一萬三千人到五萬人，台灣四大醫院一開始提供的「聚焦超音波」服務，則是一種非侵入性治療，整合神經科、神經影像科、神經外科等團隊，為原發性顫抖症以及巴金森病的患者提供另一種選擇，這項技術全名為 Magnetic Resonance-guided Focused Ultrasound，縮寫為 MRgFUS；中文全名為「經顱磁振導航超音波聚焦手術」，簡稱「神波刀」。

我向周遭關心病情的朋友提到，我即將進行神波刀治療，之後應該就不會再顫抖了。他們聽到之後皆是一臉茫然，因為巴金森病只有越來越嚴重，沒聽說過會好起來的，更何況這還是常見的老人疾病呢？！

至於我們為什麼將這個手術取名為「神波刀」？中國醫藥大學附設醫院神經部蔡崇豪主任表示，約在2018年將此技術送衛生機關審查之時，特別將「經顱磁振導航聚焦超音波」命名為「神波刀」，這是認為「神」這個字眼有上帝的大能及祝福，也有神經系統之意；治療後顫抖立除，效果真的很神。至於「波」乃因此治療之源為聚焦式超音波。「刀」字義上有治療之意，波刀所到之處，疾病就會消失，真是簡潔有力！

神波刀的治療原理 02

在台灣，中國醫藥大學附設醫院、台大醫院等四大醫院於 2022 年 8 月開啓聚焦超音波的服務，整合了神經科、神經影像科、神經外科、放射科等多專科醫護人員的專業團隊，爲原發性顫抖症以及巴金森病的患者帶來更進階的醫療服務。我的眼光則是專注在「聚焦超音波單側丘腦燒灼術」！

2016 年，科學家以聚焦超音波燒灼人腦單側的丘腦（Thalamus）神經核，發現可改善原發性顫抖症的顫抖症狀，比例更將近有五成之多，在治療過後的四年內，療效維持不墜。

聚焦超音波的原理是在特殊定位儀器的輔助下，以高功率之超音波對體內特定深度之組織加溫；運用在腦部，則可進行神經核的燒灼，阻斷產生顫抖的神經迴路。治療時，以特製頭盔聚集 1,024 束超音波束，搭配腦部核磁共振影像之立體定位，即能以非侵入性的方式，精準燒灼腦部深處幾毫米（mm）大小的神經組織，其中磁振造影成像系統就像「神波刀」的「眼睛」，使醫師在術前及術中能夠高精度識別和瞄準病灶靶點。透過磁振造影成像之引導，為患者制定個人化的治療計劃，並且在術中以磁振造影即時監測病灶靶點溫度變化，確定能量聚焦在病灶靶點，術後並即時以磁振造影確認病灶靶區治療之後的訊號變化。

另外，此儀器可發射達一千多束超音波，藉由超音波將高能量精確聚焦深部腦組織，以達治療的效果。治療過程中，首先會用較低能量超音波聚焦到腦部病灶治療靶點，接著對患者的顫抖反應進行即時評估，包括顫抖的緩解及是否有任何非預期的反應，例如無力、麻、頭痛、頭暈、噁心、嘔吐等。當病人的顫抖減緩與確認的病灶靶點正確無誤後,再逐漸提高超音波能量,使其能精準的消融病灶,讓患者在術後顫抖的情況,可以立即得到改善。

神波刀治療過程不需開腦,不需全身麻醉,大幅降低了感染與出血的風險。這個術式運用磁振造影以及高能量超音波,沒有輻射,不需要開顱且無植入物。

常見的副作用是,約有 20% 的受試者會出現短暫性的頭暈、噁心、嘔吐、無力、麻、頭痛或是步態異常,而上述情況多半在術後追蹤一至三個月內都會消失,根據四年的追蹤文獻報告,神波刀燒灼術改善原發性顫抖症,其效果到第四年的時候仍然改善 60% 甚至 70%,且無持續性的副作用。

美國和台灣的衛生主管機關,相繼於 2016 年及 2017 年先後核准聚焦超音波用於治療原發性顫抖症之患者。目前這項治療尚未納入健保給付,接受治療的病患需自費,各家醫療院所收費均不一樣;住院療程基本上是三至四天,入院後接受治療前檢查並安排聚焦超音波治療,治療隔日即可出院，之後再回門診追蹤治療。

聚焦超音波在巴金森的適應症更加廣泛，繼 2018 年美國食藥署通過「聚焦超音波燒灼單側基底核（Basal Ganglia）可治療巴金森患者藥物反應不佳之顫抖」後，2021 年 11 月，美國食藥署又核准了聚焦超音波燒灼蒼白球（Globus Pallidus）治療巴金森的異動症（Dyskinesia）。在這些核准之前，只有兩個醫療機構報告的小規模臨床試驗，認為聚焦超音波進行單側蒼白球燒灼術（Unilateral Pallidus）可改善巴金森患者的動作併發症（Motor Complication），其中包含：斷電現象減少三～四成左右、異動症改善四～五成左右。此外，Insightec 公司自 2017 年就啟動了國際臨床試驗（PD006；國際試驗案號：NCT03319485），研究聚焦超音波蒼白球燒灼術在巴金森的療效，受試者收案地點包含美國、英國、以色列、加拿大、日本、韓國及台灣。雖然正式的試驗結果尚未發表，但根據 Insightec 公司提供給美國食藥署的內部分析資料，試驗結果發現：約七成的受試者對蒼白球燒灼術有治療反應；經過十二個月後，整體減少了約三～四成的斷電現象與異動症。

根據這令人振奮的試驗初步報告，美國食藥署於 2021 年 11 月核准了聚焦超音波單側蒼白燒灼術用於中重度巴金森病的治療，此舉更加確立了該項技術在巴金森臨床治療上的重要性，期待各大醫院的跨團隊聚焦超音波治療啟動後，能為原發性顫抖症及巴金森病患者，提供免於開刀的新治療。

至於每位病患是否適合執行此技術，建議仍須前往神經部門診，經動作障礙醫師評估後再作適當安排 [2]。

這裡面提到的「導航」或「經顱磁振導航」，指的就是 MRI 磁振造影機，磁力共振（MRI）掃描有別於 X 光檢查或 CT 電腦掃描，它並沒有輻射，對人體的影響亦大大減低。

磁力共振（MRI）掃描可多角度拍攝身體內部器官的組織和結構，讓醫生可以看到患者腦部、骨骼、心臟等全身的清晰影像。

MRI 檢查大多需時二十至六十分鐘，無痛亦無需麻醉，不涉及電離輻射，無吸收輻射之憂。這台 MRI 就宛如一台隧道機，病人躺著，滑進隧道，就可以做檢查。而腦部磁力共振掃描可診斷的疾病例如腦部炎症、腫塊、結構問題，亦可診斷大腦內出血、大腦血管動脈瘤、中風、創傷性腦損傷等。

磁振造影（Magnetic Resonance Imaging，MRI）的優點除了不須要侵入人體，即可得人體各種結構組織之任意截面剖面圖，且可獲取其它眾多的物理參數訊息。MRI 檢查在全世界十幾年來至今尚未發現對人體有任何副作用。它不會產生游離輻射，對人體不具侵襲性，故不論使用多少次，都不會像 X 光等傳統檢查方法，對人體造成輻射傷害，且可多方向掃描，提供三度空間影像，又有高對比的解像力等優點[3]。

最新型之 MRI 機種（Signa MRI Infinity Excite）其成像速度更快，影像解析度更高，提供更快速、細微、清晰的高畫質影像，任何病痛將無所遁形，幫助臨床醫師，無微不至地照顧大眾的健康,達到早期診斷、預防保健的目的。

其中核磁共振成像系統就像神波刀的「眼睛」,讓醫生能夠高精度識別和瞄準靶點。通過核磁共振成像引導,為患者制定個人化的治療計劃,並且即時監測溫度,術後即時確認療效。

神波刀治療顫抖的實例

03

神波刀最早是用在治療原發性顫抖症病人。2019 年，74 歲的 C 先生按照預定流程，準備迎接他生命中最重大的轉折點，陪他一起經歷整個轉折過程的人，除了親愛的兒女們，還有一組陣容完整的醫護團隊，包括神經內、外科醫生、神經放射科醫師、研究人員以及護理人員，每位醫護人員早在 C 先生住院前，就已擬定完整的治療評估計畫，務求能讓 C 先生獲得滿意的治療效果。

C 先生是一位罹患原發性顫抖已逾十年的病人，這種神經退化疾病定不是致命的急症，但雙手逐漸嚴重的顫抖卻會讓日常生活造成極大的不便，舉凡拿筆寫字、舉杯喝水、與人握手等一般人覺得再容易不過的小事，皆無法順利完成,不少病人因此產生自卑心理,出現社交退縮甚至憂鬱等症狀。

經過許多臨床研究,神經醫學專家發現,只要以低能量的超音波束聚焦於病人的一側丘腦腹中核(Ventral Intermediate Nucleus of Thalamaus),病人對側手部的顫抖便可獲得明顯改善。

這項治療的優點是病人不必承受開刀的風險,整個治療過程保持清醒,更不需全身或半身麻醉,對於大部分罹患此病的長者而言,確實是一項極為合適的治療方式。因為在全球許多國家已被證明這種「經顱磁振導航聚焦超音波」(台灣簡稱神波刀)使用於臨床的安全性及有效性,美國食品藥物管理局(FDA)於 2016 年 7 月核准神波刀治療原發性顫抖,台灣衛生福利部也於 2017 年 11 月核准國內病人使用,在眾多因素的配合下,C 先生成為中國醫藥大學附設醫院首位接受神波刀治療的病人。

治療過程中,醫療團隊透過精準的計算和操控 1,024

個超音波探頭能量，確認 C 先生左側丘腦腹中核病灶所在，當給予的超音波能量到達一定程度時，C 先生驚訝地發現自己的右手顫抖症狀竟然消失。治療完畢後，他順手拿起身旁的杯子自在地喝下一口水，並且感動地表示，自己終於可以再用手拿起杯子喝水了！而這一刻，他竟等了十幾年……[4]。

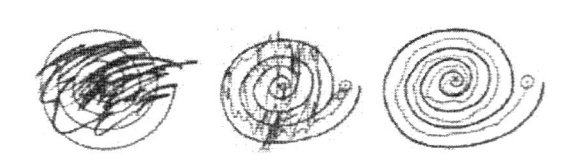

上圖由左至右，分別為 C 先生治療前、治療中及治療後，用右手拿筆所畫之螺旋圖。

| 肆、曙光出現—神波刀、聚焦超音波 |

我的神波刀治療經過

04

　　就診初期，我已經透過門診醫師開立的診斷評估，由神經內科小組助理人員作相關動作的評量，等到神波刀治療日期安排確定後，神經內科小組助理人員再度要求我來做更深入的評量，這項大約二小時的肌肉伸展與動作和思維的評量，包含在頭部、手臂和腳部肌肉的部位裝上感測鈕扣，測試肌肉表層對於電流的反應；步行在有電壓的地毯上，記錄兩腳的步行壓力大小；以及各項肢體動作的錄像等。以便做出術前及術後的改善差異對照。此外還有很重要的一個步驟就是MRI－治療之前病灶的定位，藉由磁振造影來作確定（部分內容摘錄自台大醫院巴金森症醫療中心簡介「神波刀～聚焦超音波!!」)

　　治療前定位是聚焦超音波燒灼術的成功與否的關鍵,大幅取決於燒灼位置的精準度及超音波能量的聚焦度。因此在接受治療前,患者須先接受腦部核磁共振(MRI)影像檢查,確認腦內神經結構與血管走向等資訊,同時也須接受頭骨電腦斷層影像檢查,確認顱骨密度(Skull Den sity Ratio,SDR)是否適合接受這樣的手術。實際做法是,藉由頭部外固定的立體定位頭架提供座標指引,讓醫師定位出丘腦中某一特定的為小區域「腹中間核」(Ventral Intermediate Nucleus of Thalamaus,Vim)的位置。由於 Vim 介面中,神經核與丘腦其他神經核之間並無天然分界,因此會使用正常人的腦部結構常模作為測試的基準點。而顱骨骨質密度檢測則是術前的最後一關,根據統計,顱骨骨質密度大於 0.4 者,更適合接受聚焦超音波的治療,需術前做腦部電腦斷層做判斷。MRI 進行大約 40 分鐘至 50 分鐘不等,只作頭部,身體其他部位沒有,不用麻醉也不用服用顯影劑,感覺很輕鬆自在(部

肆、曙光出現─神波刀、聚焦超音波

分內容摘錄自台大醫院巴金森症醫療中心簡介「神波刀～聚焦超音波！！」）。

　　接著是進行神波刀的書面說明書，也預先告知頭髮要剃光、要帶彈性襪和紙尿褲辦理住院。紙尿褲是因手術前後長達四小時，若中途要下來尿尿會不方便。而穿彈性絲襪是為了防止一些人腿部的血液輸送不順暢，造成血栓。事後我並沒有尿在紙尿褲上，但有更深入一層的防範也是必要的。

　　然後是安排住進病房，準備迎接明日神波刀的治療。

　　住院第一天，醫療助理會來到病房確定所預備的東西是否完備。蔡崇豪主任帶著六、七位醫師及實習醫師前來，確定我畫圈圈、手腳顫動、語言表達等的病癥作錄影，並確定停止服用巴金森及其他藥物。

　　第二天一早，第一件事是再度剃髮，要剃到用剃刀摸不出髮根的光滑程度才行。待穿上襪子、紙尿褲後，由操作神波刀設備的醫師為我戴上合金做成的頭盔，樣子像是一頂皇冠。它的功用在確保頭部的位置，不會隨著患者肩頸移動而偏離要施作神波刀的位置，畢竟這個位置只是小小的一個點，而腦部密密麻麻的職司幾十億個思維和指令，每一個點都有它的功用，容不得絲毫偏差。

除了戴上頭盔，還要為頭盔拴緊螺絲，這會造成頭殼挎緊的刺痛，所以醫師會在頭皮要拴緊螺絲的部位，施打小劑量的麻醉藥。這是整個過程中，唯一會有痛感的地方。

於是，我就這樣戴著頭盔，坐著輪椅，由病房被推送來到一間特殊的房間，裡面主要是一台極大的機器，很像是一台更大台的 MRI，而且還有一個監控室，裡面已約有十名專家坐鎮，大家穿著醫師白袍，準備見證整個過程。

手術室開始忙碌起來。有人檢查監視設備，有人檢查機台的水、電力等。而我則是要在頭盔裡戴上矽膠材質的緊實帽子，有點像猶太教男士配戴的小黑帽。其功用是在神波刀聚焦發熱於病灶時，**讓冰水在帽內流動**，

| 肆、曙光出現－神波刀、聚焦超音波 |

藉以降溫，以免腦部承受不住高溫而受損。

我躺在神波刀的手術台上，因為要施作超音波，怕音波會令我感到難受，所以兩耳戴上耳塞。然後技師在我手裡安放一個按鈕開關，表示若覺得不舒服就按鈕，控制室就會知道……。上述種種的貼心設計，我其實通通用不到。因為事實上整個過程就是躺著而已。

「神波刀」聚焦超音波的原理，是在特殊定位儀器的輔助下，以高功率超音波對體內特定深度的組織加溫；運用在腦部，則可進行神經核的燒灼，阻斷產生顫抖的神經迴路，治療時，以特製頭盔聚集 1,024 束超音波束，搭配腦部磁振造影的立體定位，即能以非侵入性的方式，精準燒灼腦部深處幾毫米大小的神經組織 [5]。

作為病人的我，事前也不知道神波刀是如何操作的，第一輪大約十幾分鐘的時間，聽到頭頂上有水流的聲音，耳朵裡聽到的則是「的～～的～～」高音的敲擊聲，然後退出神波刀機器的隧道口。一堆人從監控室來到我身旁，我感覺雙手還在顫抖著呢，就連腳也微微地發抖。

這些人各忙各的，有人檢查我的頭盔，有人觀察冰水系統……，我只聽到蔡主任以十足堅定的語氣告訴我：「現在，要再加強一些哦！」

　　緊接著，「的～～的～～」、「咚～～咚～～」的敲擊聲更急促，更尖銳。只是經過了第二輪、第三輪、第四輪的治療後，我的右手還是在顫抖。這時，肩頸部反射出酸、痛、麻的不適感。我這時才明白，原來巴金森病會造成肩頸的痠痛，只有在平躺的過程中，才會感覺到。

　　神波刀的整個進行過程，病患在神波刀機台上會先接受低能量的聚焦超音波，刺激預設的 Vim 區域，並慢慢提升至高能量。在階梯式推進的過程中，每次刺激會造成腦部微小區域的短暫升溫，透過溫度顯像儀，醫護人員便能隔空感測超音波能量對於腦部組織的升溫效果，再逐步定位測試與提高能量。這此一過程中，醫護人員也會進入監控室為病患進行顫抖症狀評估，當確立測試區域能達到最大程度的症狀改善時，便施以最高能量燒灼，將腦部組織溫度提升至治療溫度（約攝氏 56 度上下），藉此達到永久性的燒灼 6。

待到了第五輪的治療，我確實感覺到音波變得更強大，頭頂壓力更強了，甚至連肩膀的痠痛變得更明顯，畢竟躺久了，總想要變換姿勢，但即便如此，還是建議不能亂動，所以我只好繼續忍耐著……。大約再過十五分鐘後，機器停止運轉，我又再次退出隧道，咦？！我這時發現手不抖了，腳也不抖了！空氣瞬間凝滯，我全身竟然都不再顫抖了！

下了機台，我立刻伸出右手，伸直五個指頭，正面瞧瞧，反面看看，再伸直給蔡主任看，我不禁高喊著：「都不會抖了！」為了怕暈眩，而且此刻急著想卸下頭盔，因為頭盔現在變成箍緊頭部的累贅。所以就在助理人員的安排下，怕我會暈眩站不穩，因此再度坐上輪椅，在蔡主任引導下，跟著做幾個檢視巴金森病的手部及腳部動作，然後問我現在的感覺如何？我回答說：「我現在都不抖了，看來手術很成功，值得喝采！」現場的其他醫護人員、技師、實習醫師們也全都不自主地鼓掌起來，現場頓時有如慶功場面一般！

當卸下頭盔、卸下頭部矽膠小帽，我知道治療成功了！心裡有如卸下萬斤重擔般開心。

台大醫院影像醫學部有繪製「神波刀治療流程」，內容淺顯易懂，我在此摘錄下來供各界人士參考。

神波刀治療流程：

第一步－患者準備：治療前，進行電腦斷層及磁振造影掃描，以便評估是否適合治療。

治療當天，術前剃光頭髮，並局部麻醉以固定立體定向框架。患者仰臥在治療床上，頭部置於「神波刀」頭盔內，並以冷卻水在頭皮周圍循環降溫。

第二步－治療計畫：通過結合術前和術中磁振造影來制訂治療計劃，確定治療靶點。

第三步－靶點驗證：治療時先使用較低能量超音波聚焦到治療靶點，再逐漸提高能量，對患者反應進行即時評估。

第四步—開始治療：將高能量超音波把能量精確匯聚到靶點，並以磁振造影持續即時監測靶區溫度變化。逐漸將靶點溫度升高至攝氏 60 度左右，以造成靶組織的熱消融。

第五步—評估（治療結束後）：採用畫螺旋線或其他測試方法來評估顫抖的改善情況。最後一次超音波治療後，掃描磁振造影影像以確認消融區域。

---

1. 見台大校訊 1542 期「顫抖不再」文，及網路搜尋：中國醫藥大學附設醫院「經顱磁振導航聚焦超音波」文。
2. 台大醫院巴金森病醫療中心簡介「神波刀～聚焦超音波！！」
3. 中國醫藥大學附設醫院「經顱磁振導航聚焦超音波（神波刀）簡介」。
4. 中國醫藥大學附設醫院神經科呂明桂醫師、陳睿正醫師、蔡崇豪主任撰〈匯聚千束超音波神奇的力量，神波刀成功治療原發性顫抖〉，2020 年 4 月 15 日，《中國醫訊》第 192 期。
5. 「顫抖不再」 台大醫院認識 （神波刀） 記者會 ，《台大校訊》第 1542 期。
6. 台大醫院巴金森病醫療中心簡介「神波刀～聚焦超音波！！」

伍、治療後……

術後當下的感受 01

　　離開神波刀的治療機台後,我再次被送回病房並且睡了兩個多小時的午覺。醫護人員事先有說,神波刀治療後,由於腦部受到燒灼的耗能影響,會出現身體虛弱的現象,所以需要更多的睡眠來補充體力。而這次的午睡,其實是被兩腿的抽筋所驚醒。我已有十多年沒有在睡眠或登山時腳抽筋,如今兩腿都抽筋,感覺很奇特。接下,來我從病房走到茶水間倒水來喝,路程大約二十多公尺遠,這時走起路來,感覺右腳跟不上步伐,會被拖著走,而且右腳腳尖還會偏離正常位置。

　　在前述「神波刀的醫治原理」該章節中,我曾引用台大醫院巴金森病醫療中心的介紹,文中表示「約佔

20%的受試者會出現副作用（指神波刀），多數是短暫的頭暈、噁心、無力、麻、頭痛或步態異常。一般在術後追一至三個月內會消失。」2021年7月在《神經醫學雜誌》（Movement-Disorde）上發表的一個第二期臨床研究BEST-FUS Trial 2指出，為原發性顫抖患者進行雙側丘腦聚焦超音波燒灼術，仍可獲得療效；但追蹤三個月後，10人之中有7個人會出現輕微副作用，例如口齒不清、吞嚥困難、步態不穩等。

我在住院第三天，也就是神波刀治療後的次日，當蔡主任帶著四位醫師來到我跟前巡診時，我也有向醫師陳述上述異狀。此後兩週，累計我術後的異常狀況計有：

一、步態異常，只有右邊單側，右腳會有跟不上左腳步距的狀況。

二、右手上臂的肌肉仍然向內緊縮，右手指力也不如左手。

三、口齒言語表達上，使用字彙不夠清晰周延，用詞簡化且聲調低沉，令聆聽者感覺怪怪的。

四、無法走過長的距離,每次步行約八百公尺就是極限了,然後要坐著休息才行。

所幸這些狀況,都在之後三到五個月內陸續改善,最明顯的就是語言表達的能力在三個月內達到滿意的狀態,例如唱歌,我覺得自己應該是唱得不錯吧,哈哈!從剛開始時會有一些咬字不清楚,來到五個月後能夠完整地唱完一首歌,感覺真棒。至於噁心、嘔吐、麻、頭痛的狀況,我都沒有發生過,走路也可以越走越遠。

治療後不再服藥,也沒有服藥的理由!

蔡主任也安排了定期回診之外,由評量小組的人員來為我做術後的評量,同樣也是在近兩個小時內作十幾樣的檢測,另外還安排了 MRI,確定病灶靶區在治療之後的訊號變化。我在治療過後半年的某次回診中,蹲上蹲下,腳跟和腳尖著地的動作,越做越快,我對蔡主任回應說:「I Feel Better & Better!」看到蔡主任露出了笑容,我也不自覺的開懷大笑起來。

雖然不適的症狀在自然消退,但我的右腳還是有一點跟不上左腳的步距，右手臂肌肉緊縮的問題，還是有些影響觀瞻，舉動看起來怪怪的。剛巧我遇上中醫師深諳針灸和「小針刀」療法，主要是用淺淺的針刺肌肉的筋膜部位，鬆解肌肉的筋膜；又到泰國旅遊時，接受「槌筋」式的按摩，用木槌敲打筋絡。結果這兩者對我的手部和腳步都起到積極的作用，上臂肌肉緊縮感消失，右腳跟不上左腳的狀況也不存在，若真要說兩手和兩腳的差異，就只有在提行李箱，雙手負重時略有一些差異，一般情況下是完全看不出有何差異。

總結神波刀治療的七大優勢：

一、無輻射。

二、無須開顱。

三、無植入物。

四、無須麻醉，患者在整個治療過程中清醒。

五、熱燒熔精準 + 溫度可控。

六、術後感染出血風險極低。

七、術後快速恢復正常生活。

所以，它是極安全又立即有效的一次性治療。在我前後治療的三天裡，並未有家人陪同，出院後自行搭車離去，來到熟悉的早餐店吃蛋餅、喝豆漿，總之，一切就是輕鬆自在。

一年半過去了……

02

　　神波刀治療後,大約一年的時間裡,我報名參加了一場萬人健走活動,在山區走大馬路,感覺有點起伏但幅度不大,總長距離是六公里,我走到終點前已感到心力用盡,因此大約六公里是我的底線。不料到一年半後的現在,因為腳的施力比較強,且上下樓梯的步伐比較自然,現在一天包含上下階梯,能夠走一萬八千步。以前對於爬坡視為畏途,如今走台中市大坑山區的步道,上坡坡度大約三十度,感覺也不構成問題,下坡則更顯輕鬆,不會再有精力耗盡的感覺。

　　唱歌時的咬字,在治療後三個月時,或許有點咬字不夠精準,如今即使碰到快節奏的歌曲,也很順利唱好。

只是在跳舞上,遇上快節奏的步伐,有時會自然反應把三步併成兩步,結果造成步伐錯亂!我想,腿部的神經還需要假以時日鍛鍊,應該越來越好。

我曾試著小跑步,比如走過十字路口,遇到燈號快要截止時,會小跑步加速跑,但是不能夠持續一直跑下去,主要是快跑時,右腳步伐協調略有落差,猶如在跳舞時,會跟不上快節奏的步伐一樣。

右手拿湯匙或叉子送食物放進嘴巴裡時,原先會有傾斜而把食物提前掉落的情況,現在已能穩定進食,湯匙或食物也不會再掉落了。

臉部的表情也徹底改變了,原本很嚴肅沉默的臉,變得有笑容而且柔軟,看過我前後的人也都認同。

我樂觀地認為,腦中的多巴胺分泌一旦來到正常狀態,大腦所下達學習的指令,會促使神經迴路再次增強嘗試的動機。將學習到的資訊反覆輸出練習,動作自然會越來越好。

神經學當中的「赫布理論」(Hebbian Theory)曾提

到,「突觸前神經元向突觸後神經元的持續重複的刺激,可以導致突觸傳遞效能的增加」。或者說「由對神經元的重複刺激,使得神經元之間的突觸強度增加」,所以持續動作可以改善不夠完美的動作,包括跑步和跳舞也是一樣。

所以神波刀的治療模式,並不是一種「截斷」神經的方式,它是掃除路障然後「重組」已經退化的組織,讓多巴胺神經細胞再度分泌正常濃度的多巴胺,進而去除巴金森病狀,藉由神經元的反覆刺激,讓身體動作回復正常狀態。

感謝 03

我以往認為,一旦確定罹患巴金森病,病情並不會隨著服用藥物而停止或受到控制,對巴金森病狀的治療,通常是左多巴藥物或其他相關藥物來輔助,用藥時間過長就可能帶來副作用,例如病人會有異常的肢體扭動(異動症),因此,精準穩定藥物在血液中的濃度,非常重要。

除了藥物治療外,還有一種稱為腦深層刺激 DBS 的治療方式。手術的流程是將細長的電極導線置於病人腦部,並在胸鎖骨附近(類似心律調節器的安裝位置)植入發生器並與導線相連。透過電流來調節腦內錯誤的訊息,藉此改善病人的症狀。但是腦深層刺激手術仍不能夠完全治療巴金森病。

| 伍、治療後…… |

在我身上的神波刀治療,可謂開啟了醫療界對巴金森病治療的一扇窗。

神波刀治療之後,顫抖會立刻停止,雖然可能會有伴隨口齒表達不清,步履不穩及噁心等症狀,但是這些會隨著時間而慢慢淡化,甚至隨著動作的增強而改善。

對於神波刀改善或停止下墜式的病況,改善體適能狀況,改進生活動作的不便,重拾生活上的自尊心,去除對藥物的依賴,去除死亡的陰影,在我身上都有著立竿見影的顯著效果。

在我進行神波刀治療的隔天,一群實習醫師來觀察我的病情,我簡短地告訴他們:「你們選擇了正確的科別,神經科加上神波刀,可以幫助千千萬萬的病人和家屬們免除痛苦!」

在我到中國醫藥大學附設醫院的神經科回診之中,我也數次不自覺地握起蔡崇豪醫師的雙手,不斷地向他「道謝」,表達自己無限的敬意與感謝。

目前核磁共振引導聚焦超音波治療系統,已在多個國家獲得核准使用於臨床治療，例如美國、歐洲、以色列、加拿大、韓國、日本、中國、泰國和澳大利亞等。

神波刀適用於小範圍病灶的非侵入性治療，國內外也發展並進行多項研究中，如控制神經性疼痛、針對特定器官或腫瘤投遞藥物、輔助打開血腦屏障，協助腫瘤化療治療成效、血栓溶解、精神相關疾病如憂鬱症等。神波刀的應用廣泛，又有微創及精準之優點，因此其角色必越發重要[1]。

目前全球有超過六百萬人罹患巴金森病，而得到神波刀醫療訊息的人數僅僅只有少數，當然，是否需要神波刀治療或是否適用其他治療方式，還是要看醫師的評估與判斷。然而神波刀完全治癒我的巴金森病，這是千真萬確的事實，我把自己幸運的醫療經歷公諸於世，期望神波刀能降福在有需要的病人身上，改善大家的生活品質，擁有平安、健康、幸福、快樂的美好下半場人生。

---

1. 「顫抖不再」台大醫院認識（神波刀）記者會，《台大校訊》第1542期。

CONTENTS

Author's Preface   94
Origin······   98

CHAPTER 1 | On Set

01. The origin of my Parkinson's disease   100
02. My Parkinson's Disease Status   107

CHAPTER 2 | What is Parkinson's disease?

01. How is it different from Parkinson's syndrome?   116
02. Typical external motor symptoms of Parkinson's disease   128
03. Parkinson's disease may cause mental and neurological disorders   133
04. Parkinson's disease and sleep disorders   136

CHAPTER 3 | The brain—The center for the onset of Parkinson's disease

01. Cause of Parkinson's disease   140
02. Diagnosis of Parkinson's disease   145
03. Drug treatment of Parkinson's disease   151
04. Deep brain stimulation surgery—DBS   160

CHAPTER 4 | Dawn appears—Magnetic Resonance-guided Focused Ultrasound (MRgFUS)

01. The origin and naming of MRgFUS   164
02. The healing principle of MRgFUS   168
03. Cases of using MRgFUS to treat tremors   177
04. My MRgFUS treatment experience   181

CHAPTER 5 | After MRgFUS treatment

01. How you feel immediately after surgery   194
02. Current situation one and a half years after MRgFUS treatment   200
03. Conclusion   204

I Feel So Good !

I was born in an ordinary family, and grew up with a balanced development of physical fitness, intellectual development, and habits. After middle age, I have no problems such as high blood pressure, blood lipids, heart disease, and uric acid. After reaching the age of sixty, I suddenly noticed that my right hand would tremble. As time passes year after year, the trembling became more and more obvious, and then my right leg also started to tremble. To sum up, this kind of trembling is not just a problem of shaking frequency, but also the uncontrollable anxiety that accompanies the displacement of the muscles in the hands and legs.

My grandfather, father, and I are all eldest sons, and they all also suffer from tremors. My father wasn't diagnosed with Parkinson's until he was 90. So I initially thought that Parkinson's disease was just a condition that causes trembling hands. With the accelerated progress of my disease, and with

/Preface

the improvement of modern mobile phone query functions, I was able to obtain very detailed information about Parkinson's disease. When I finally learned of my illness, and that it would continue to deteriorate to the point of paralyzing me in my hospital bed or even causing my early death, the fear and anxiety in my heart were as great as a boulder weighing me down.

My fear and anxiety come from Parkinson's disease. Although it is a neurological disease that is easily acquired by the elderly, it has always been controlled mainly with drugs or rehabilitation methods, but it cannot stop or suppress the disease. The patient will deteriorate over time. Aggravating the condition, patients must have in-depth interactions with doctors during medical treatment, and patients and their families must be extremely patient and considerate. This is an irreversible disease. What I have always felt worried and anxious about is, in today's world of advanced technology, why is there

Emerging from the Shadows of Parkinson's Disease

no cure for this disease ?

I learned about the function of Shenbo Knife from the internet. I asked the doctor about it. About half a year later, the doctor told me that I could undergo the medical treatment of the Shenbo Knife. I later learned that Shenbo Knife can control tremors, but Parkinson's patients need detailed evaluation because the pathogenesis of Parkinson's disease is extremely complex. A medical team is needed to observe, analyze, and propose medical strategies to help the doctor make a precise diagnosis and treatment. I happen to be suitable for Shenbo Knife treatment, so among the many patients in Parkinson's, I am considered an extremely lucky person.

Now, I don't take any medication. I occasionally go hiking with friends or take a day trip for a walk. I no longer tremble, my muscle soreness has disappeared, and I have become the same me ! When most people suffer from Parkinson's

/Preface

disease, their movements become smaller and smaller, so the chance of being able to write down a detailed description of the disease is low. I picked up a pen to write down the entire process from the state of recovery from the disease, which can be regarded as a way of giving back to medical progress. I would like to sincerely thank the entire medical team at China Medical University Hospital for their patient efforts and precise medical treatment, which enabled me to witness the full picture of Parkinson's disease, break out of it, and regain a new life.

This book was published thanks to the employees of Jiuyang Computer Information Co., Ltd. for their quick editing and correction. I would also like to thank those who care about my condition. I would like to respond happily：I Feel So Good !

Chang, C. David

Origin······

I was born in February 1958. I will be 67 years old when the book is published this year, 2025.

I was first diagnosed with Parkinson's disease in 2020 at the age of 61 at China Medical University Hospital in Taichung. In October 2022, under the operation of MRgFUS medical team led by Director Chon-Haw Tsai of the Department of Neurology at China Medical University Hospital, Shenbo Knife-Magnetic Resonance-guided Focused Ultrasound (MRgFUS) treatment was carried out.

From the moment I stepped off the operating table, I knew that my Parkinson's disease had been completely removed from my body !

It has been a year and two years now, and I've gone from having my body movements gradually deteriorate to living a happy, normal life. Before undergoing MRgFUS treatment, I knew that Parkinson's disease will gradually decline, that the physical condition is irreversible, and that there is no cure, but I can walk more than 18,000 steps today. I proudly confessed to the doctor on the day I went back to the clinic：「I Feel Better & Better ！ I can already declare MRgFUS completely cured my Parkinson's disease ！」

Chapter 1
On Set

The origin of my Parkinson's disease

When I was 30, my father was 60. My father lives an extremely disciplined life. He does not smoke or drink, does not play cards or socialize, does not eat spicy food, and does not drink tea or coffee. He has regular health checkups. Except for low blood pressure, very light sleep, and occasional constipation, the health check report values are all very healthy. He goes to bed early and gets up early. He walks to the neighborhood at 05：30 every morning. He returns home for a breakfast of bread and milk around 7 o'clock. In the community of civil servants where my father lived, there were very few people as extremely disciplined and healthy as he was. When I was 30 years old, because I had a stable job and had more

Chapter 1. On Set

time to pay attention to my family, I accidentally discovered that my father's left hand would tremble. For example, when eating, his left hand was holding a bowl. His right hand was about to pick up food, the part where the fingers hold the edge of the bowl, will shake up and down. Also, when pointing out something, the hands will be gestured in front of the chest. You can see that the fingers of the left hand are shaking at an abnormal and high frequency.

My father explained that this is a hereditary hand tremor syndrome, but it will not affect health because there are no adverse effects other than hand tremors. My father retired at the age of 65 and often travels between Taiwan and Zhejiang Province, China, because his father, my grandfather, lived in Zhejiang. The reason why hand tremors are hereditary in the family is because my father said that his father had hand tremors since he was young, and he was very healthy and had never seen a doctor for illness in his life.

As far as I can remember, my grandfather always had a smile on his face when he met people. He had a thin and dark physique. He often hid his wrists in his sleeves. He also had a large appetite. Sometimes he could eat 8 boiled eggs in one meal. He lived to the age of 98 and died in a natural state.

My father has always looked healthy. When my grandfather was alive, he also looked extremely healthy. His hands and feet were flexible and there were no signs of decline. The trembling hands are one of those things that just naturally become an everyday part of life. In 2006, I took my father to Xitou Scenic Area for a hiking trip. There were some hills along the way. We walked for about two and a half hours. When my father was eating, his hands were trembling obviously. The amplitude is quite noticeable. Looking at his uncontrollable hands, will it affect health and lifespan ? So I began to search for literature from various sources, eager to explain this problem.

However, at this time, my father still insisted that this hand tremors inherited in the family. Everyone in the family lived a long life. By that time, as children, we have realized that what was described in the literature was obviously Parkin-

Chapter 1. On Set

son's disease.

At the beginning of 2019, my father accidentally fell during his morning walk. A medical doctor near my home reminded me that a fall in the elderly is a warning sign and should not be taken lightly. It is necessary to go to a large hospital for a complete physical examination. So we chose to go to Taichung Veterans General Hospital for detailed examinations in various departments related to motor neurology. The neurology department immediately diagnosed my father with Parkinson's disease, but because other symptoms were not obvious, he was not prescribed any medication. It means that the doctor thinks the condition is not serious.

My father was already ninety years old at the time. Apart from trembling hands, leaning forward slightly, and walking in small steps, there were no other abnormal symptoms that could be detected by the naked eye. I suddenly remembered that I myself had experienced inexplicable shaking of my fingers several times, so I asked the doctor to help me evaluate it. The doctor asked me to do a few actions, including squatting, walking back and forth, and moving my fingers. The conclusion was : there was nothing abnormal.

In the spring of 2020, my father fell again while hiking in the morning. The cause of the fall was completely blank in his mind. He didn't know how he fell, and he didn't know what happened after the fall. In the following days, his physical condition, if you were to express it in terms of a coordinate curve, it would be a downward curve off a cliff. He does not eat or drink, has incontinence of urine and feces, has weak eyesight, lies in bed all day, and refuses to communicate.

My sister and I first sent him to Taichung Veterans General Hospital. Then transferred him to a local hospital for hospitalization and long-term care. During this period, he took the doctor's prescription for "Amanda" (a drug for Parkinson's disease), twe pills a day. Then he contracted pneumonia and took pneumonia medicine at the same time. Except for sitting on the bedside to talk to people, he spent the rest of the time in bed and sleeping.

In the last few dozen days, respirators and blood oxygen

Chapter 1. On Set

monitoring are necessary. More than five months after being admitted to the hospital, my father passed away naturally while sitting and resting at the age of ninety-two.

During my father's funeral, I held a microphone in my hand to express my thoughts about my father to the guests. Later, my cousin asked me curiously, why my hands kept shaking？I immediately answered him without hesitation, I have Parkinson's disease.

At that time, I had not been diagnosed by a doctor. My situation was the same as my father's. At the same time, in recent Sundays, I served as a master of ceremonies in church, and I also had to hold a microphone in one hand and hold the ritual program in my other hand to announce. Sometimes, the trembling of my right hand is like uncontrollable shaking. The only pause state is to use my non-trembling left hand to press the shaking right hand. After pressing it for a few seconds, my right hand will stop shaking. This is my initial situation.

I noticed that my right foot also began to tremble. When I stood, my right foot would involuntarily retract inward and lean toward my left foot. Then my body's center of gravity would be on the left side. In this way, my right foot would extend from my thigh to my knee, causing some trembling. The difference between the trembling of the right hand and the right foot is that the fingers and tips of the right hand can clearly be trembled, while the trembling of the right foot is less obvious. The biggest difference is that the trembling of the thigh is short-lived. At first, the tremor in my right hand was more obvious. After a while, about half a year later, the above-mentioned changes in my right foot appeared.

| Chapter 1.On Set |

My Parkinson's Disease Status

02

Shortly after my father passed away, I determined to find a cure for my own illness !

I'm an officer in a well-known society in central Taiwan. This society has established a "Health Care Committee" and invites the most famous doctors and experts in the medical field to hold regular "health lectures" to provide entrepreneurs and their family members with medical care advice. In addition, the post of medical consultant has been set up so that members can have a channel to contact for consultation in case of complicated medical problems. This prevents members from having to search for the right doctor for their condition.

I received the correct treatment through the assistance of

medical consultant Dr.Wen-Yuan Lin. He is the vice president of China Medical University Hospital and the director of the Department of Family Medicine. He is very familiar with the diseases of middle-aged and elderly people. After listening to my statement, he immediately referred me to another doctor, Chon-Haw Tsai, director of the Department of Neurology of China Medical University Hospital.

Director Chon-Haw Tsai is a medical doctor, professor and dean of the medical School. He is also the attending physician of the Parkinson's Disease and Movement Disorders Department of the Department of Neurology, China Medical University Hospital, and the Asia-Pacific Executive Director of the International Parkinson's Disease and Movement Disorders Society（2017～2021）.

The first consultation took about half an hour. The doctor asked me to draw circles on a piece of paper with each hand. And asked me to point my nose with my index finger, then touched the ball in front of me, put my toes and feet on the ground, walked back and forth, etc., and then made an appointment for brain tomography, etc.

My discomfort symptoms at that time were that the muscles of my right upper arm were retracted inward. I would wake up due to muscle soreness even during sleep. In my free time, the fingers of my right hand would shake, and my right foot would shake slightly. When I wrote, my words would become smaller and smaller. However, the two functions of walking and speaking were as usual, and there was no state of discomfort.

The prescription given by the doctor at that time was:

(1) Recognition of Parkinson's disease.

(2) No brain damage or organic disease.

(3) Temporarily take half an Amanda tablet twice a day in the morning and evening.

(4) Parkinson's disease has not affected my daily life yet.

Taking Amanda tablets is effective in suppressing tremors at the beginning, but after three or four months, it cannot be completely suppressed. For example, the tremors are reduced and the amplitude of the tremors is reduced, but there are still small amount of shaking. The same is true of the feet. The amplitude of the jitter will decrease, but it will still jitter.

The contraction of the upper arm muscles was still the main complaint when I returned to the clinic. During the subsequent three and six months of follow-up visits, I noticed that my hands shake when I'm straining to poop. My feet would tremble when I urinated. It affects the urine spraying to the left and right sides, and it is impossible to fix the urine at the same point. I also practice qigong, and there is a form called squatting with the Dantian in hands. After squatting for a few seconds, the right side from the shoulder to the knee was shaking non-stop.

Once I went to the mountainous area of Qingjing Farm with my family to play. I didn't know the route clearly, so I walked further and further away. At that moment, I had a disagreement with my family, and I was anxious to get out of the unclear route. I was nervous for a while, and the right side of my body was shaking non-stop, and the tremors were severe.

Chapter 1. On Set

It was so severe that I was shocked. Another time I participated in climbing a small mountain. If I held the pole in my right hand, I would switch to my left hand because my right hands were shaking. I switched my left and right hands several times. A sharp-eyed teammate spotted it and told me it was Parkinson's disease. I felt a little bit hurt in my self-esteem after being told that. The worst situation is that there will inevitably be times when you are driving a friend, but your right hand on the steering wheel starts to shake unconsciously, and my friend will ask∶"What's wrong with your hand？"

I learned from the Internet that "Shenbo Knife" is used to treat Parkinson's disease and tremors in Taiwan, so I made a request for this treatment to Director Chon-Haw Tsai. Director Tsai explained to me the benefits of the treatment. He advised me to observe my condition for some time before making a decision.

Just between May and August of 2022, my Parkinson's disease worsened rapidly. Two Amanda tablets a day could no longer stop the tremors. The tremors could happen at any time. I've become depressed and I don't talk much. My voice has become deeper. I have choked easily when eating. Even when riding a bicycle, the right foot does not follow the inertia of pedaling and easily falls off the pedal. The strength of the hands are also gradually weakening. When holding the mug with the right hand, the shaking of the hand will cause the water in the cup to overflow, which is really distressing. I learned from the literature that Parkinson's disease will worsen, become stiff, collapse on the bed, and eventually lead to death. The shadow of fear in my heart becomes heavier and lingering.

Apart from Parkinson's disease, my physical condition is still very good. My blood pressure has always been maintained at 75 ~ 120mm-Hg (millimeters of mercury). My heart rate has always been between 70 and 80. My height is 174cm and my weight is 75Kg. I have no blood lipid problems. I have no uric acid problem. My defecation and sleeping status have always been normal. I don't smoke or drink. I only have one cup of coffee a day, and occasionally go hiking with my friends.

A whole-body PET examination was performed in 2021. Except for the discovery of small nodules on the thyroid gland in the neck, which were later confirmed to be benign by ultrasound and puncture examination, no other adverse conditions were found.

This is probably due to my optimistic personality. I always look on the bright side. However, Parkinson's disease really puts me under tremendous pressure of life and death······！！

Chapter 2
What is Parkinson's disease ?

How is it different from Parkinson's syndrome?

Parkinson's symptoms is a broader term that describes a group of movement disorder symptoms (slowness of movement, tremors, muscle stiffness, postural instability) that may be caused by a variety of conditions, including Parkinson's disease, other neurodegenerative diseases, drugs or toxins. The so-called Parkinson's disease is a progressive neurodegenerative disease. Its pathological mechanism is the massive loss of dopamine-producing neurons in the brainstem, resulting in symptoms such as slow movement, stiffness, and tremors.

Parkinson's disease, Alzheimer's disease and stroke are listed as the three major diseases of the elderly. The main characteristics are:

Chapter 2. What is Parkinson's disease?

(1) They don't show up until they reach a certain age.
(2) There is a certain high proportion.
(3) Both men and women have it.
(4) All are difficult to cure and will affect life.

Neurological diseases are the leading cause of disability, and Alzheimer's disease (dementia) and Parkinson's disease are the two most common neurological degenerative diseases in the elderly. Parkinson's disease is characterized by movement disorders, including uncontrollable resting tremor, limb stiffness, poor balance, and decreased motor function. In addition, there are a wide variety of non-motor symptoms that cause trouble in life. Some symptoms even appear long before the motor symptoms occur, such as constipation, depression, loss of smell, moving hands and feet in sleep, etc. In Taiwan, the average age at which this disease occurs is about 60 to 62 years old. The prevalence rate in this group is about 1%. The incidence of the disease in men is 1.5 times that of women. It is estimated that there are currently about 30,000 to 50,000 patients in Taiwan out of a population of 23 million.

The main pathological change in Parkinson's disease is the degeneration and death of dopamine neurons in the substantia nigra of the midbrain. The cause of movement disorders is insufficient secretion of dopamine in the brain. If the motor area of the human brain is compared to the movement command center of the whole body, the basal ganglia (This is described in Chapter 3 of this book) is like the office of the Chief of Staff. Dopamine is like the base of messengers. The command system of patients with Parkinson's disease is because the training base cannot cultivate enough messengers, resulting in disordered message transmission. Insufficient instructions prevent the command center from leading the limbs to complete daily movements. (**Note 1**)

The condition was first discovered and documented by British physician James Parkinson. Parkinson's disease is a progressive disease that gradually affects the patient's nervous system and various parts of the nervous system. Parkinson's disease mostly affects middle-aged and elderly people, but there are also cases of the disease in young adults. Patients who develop the disease before the age of 50 are called young Parkinson's disease. The course of the disease in young patients is slower and the recovery is better. (Taken from internet search: Parkinson's Disease Self-Testing and Top 5 FAQs)

According to Wikipedia, Parkinson's disease (Parkinson's disease, PD for short) is a chronic neurodegenerative disease that affects the central nervous system, mainly affecting motor nerve function. Symptoms usually appear slowly over time. The most obvious early symptom is tremors, limb stiffness, hypokinesia and gait abnormalities, and there may also be cognitive and behavioral problems. As for dementia, it is quite common in severely ill Parkinson patients. Major depressive disorder and anxiety disorders also occur in more than one-third of cases. Other symptoms that may accompany it include problems with perception, sleep, and mood.

The cause of Parkinson's disease is still unknown. It is generally believed to be related to genetic and environmental factors. People who have Parkinson's disease in their families are more likely to develop the disease. and those who are exposed to certain pesticides and have had head trauma are also at higher risk. however, those who smoke and frequently drink coffee or tea are at lower risk. The main motor symptoms of Parkinson's disease result from the death of cells in the substantia nigra of the midbrain, resulting in insufficient dopamine in the relevant brain areas of the patient. The cause of cell death is poorly understood, but it is known to be related to the process by which neuronal proteins form Lewy Bodies. Typical Parkinson's disease relies heavily on symptom diagnosis. Neuroimaging can also help rule out the possibility of other diseases.

Parkinson's disease is a movement syndrome, a collective name for several movement disorders with similar symptoms. By definition, symptoms must include bradykinesia (A decrease in voluntary movements, or a decrease in the rate and flexibility of repetitive movements, such as spontaneous finger tapping) plus one or more of the following symptoms-leadpipe, cogwheel (Meaning: when the patient is relaxed and

Chapter 2. What is Parkinson's disease？

you move his hands and feet, you will still feel resistance like a clicking gear), static tremor, and postural instability, etc. According to the above causes, they can be classified into the following four types.

(1) Idiopathic Parkinsonism

(2) Secondary Parkinsonism

(3) Heredity

(4) Parkinson-plus syndromes (Such as multiple system degeneration, corticobasal degeneration).

Parkinson's disease refers to Idiopathic Parkinsonism, meaning it has no clearly identifiable cause, and is the most common form of Parkinson's disease. In recent years, several genes have been found to be directly related to Parkinson's disease, which conflicts with the original definition based on the Idiopathic Parkinsonism. Therefore, Genetic Parkinson's disease, which has a similar course to Parkinson's disease, is also commonly referred to as Parkinson's disease. "Familial Parkinson's disease" and "sporadic Parkinson's disease" are used to distinguish between hereditary and truly unknown patient groups.

Parkinson's disease is usually classified as a motor disease. However, it can also cause other non-motor symptoms, such as sensory impairment, cognitive difficulties, and sleep disturbances. "Parkinson-plus syndromes" has other additional clinical symptoms in addition to Parkinson's symptoms. This type of disease mainly includes multiple system atrophy (MSA), progressive supranuclear palsy (PSP), corticobasal degeneration (CBD) and Dementia with Lewy bodies (DLB).

Lewy body dementia is a synuclein pathology similar to Parkinson's disease. Symptoms include hallucinations, fluctuations in attention, slowed movement, unsteady steps, or reduced motor function. Symptoms of dementia may appear in the first year before or after the onset of Parkinson's symptoms. This condition is very similar to Parkinson's disease and dementia, but the relationship between the two diseases still needs further research to clarify. They may be regarded as two separate diseases, or they may be regarded as manifestations

Chapter 2. What is Parkinson's disease？

of different aspects of one disease.

It seems that my Parkinson's disease is most likely hereditary.

In 2015, approximately 6.2 million people worldwide suffered from Parkinson's disease, causing 117,000 deaths. Parkinson's disease usually occurs in people over 60 years old, and about 1% of the elderly suffer from this disease. Men are more likely to get Parkinson's disease than women. If the disease develops in patients younger than 50 years old, it is called Early-Onset Parkinsonism（EOP）. Risk factors for Parkinson's disease that threaten patient's health include cognitive decline and dementia, swallowing disorders, geriatric onset, and more severe disease states. On the other hand, patients whose main symptom is tremors have a higher survival rate than those whose main symptoms are stiffness. People with Parkinson's disease are about twice as likely to die from Aspiration Pneumonia as healthy people. The disease is named after the British doctor James Parkinson, who published "An Essay on the Shaking Palsy" in 1817, which for the first time detailed six symptoms related to Parkinson's disease. His birthday, April 11, is also designated as World Parkinson's Day. The community groups will hold public promotion activities on this day. Tulips are the symbol of Parkinson's disease. The illness of some famous patients has raised public awareness of the disease, including People's Republic of China leader Deng Xiaoping, actor Michael J. Fox, Olympic cyclist Davis Feeney and professional boxer Muhammad Ali. (This section of the professional analysis is taken from the Internet search : Wikipedia / Parkinson's disease / Categories)

However, Parkinson's disease is easily reminiscent of Alzheimer's dementia. The two symptoms are different, but because they are diseases of the elderly. Some people suffer from both symptoms at the same time in old age. Parkinson's disease and Alzheimer's disease are both central nervous system degenerative diseases. The difference between the two is that Alzheimer's disease is the degeneration of nerve cells in the hippocampus and cerebral cortex of the brain, leading to cognitive dysfunction. Parkinson's disease is the degeneration

Chapter 2. What is Parkinson's disease?

of nerve cells in the substantia nigra of the midbrain, and its symptoms are mainly manifested in the form of movement and limb impairment. The differences between the two can be seen in the table below. (**Note 2**)

	Parkinson's disease
pathogen	Degeneration of nerve cells in the substantia nigra of the midbrain.
symptons	Symptoms are mainly in the limbs, including hand tremors, muscle stiffness, slow movements, and abnormal postures, etc.
age of onset	Most are over 50 years old, a few are under 45 years old.
treatment method	Medication is the main treatment, but surgery can also be used to improve symptoms.

| Chapter 2.What is Parkinson's disease ? |

Alzheimer's disease

Degeneration of nerve cells in the hippocampus and cerebral cortex of the brain.

Symptoms of cognitive impairment are predominant, including poor memory, abnormal speech and expression ability, loss of time concept, poor judgment, high mood swings, personality changes, and poor mobility, etc.

Most cases occur over the age of 65, but a few develop between the ages of 30 and 60 due to genetic mutations.

Medication is the main treatment, with drugs that can improve mental function such as Donepezil and Exelon being used more often.

Tabulation:Author
Source:Reprinted from the online article "Parkinson's Disease Just Started 6 Precursors,Symptom Detection,Treatment,and Life Expectancy in One Look".

Typical external motor symptoms of Parkinson's disease

Parkinson's disease has four main motor symptoms : tremors, limb stiffness, slowness of movement, and unstable posture.

Tremors are the most obvious and well-known symptom. About 30% of Parkinson's patients do not have tremors at the beginning of the disease, but as the disease progresses, most patients will gradually develop this symptom. The tremor in Parkinson's disease is usually resting tremor, that is, the limbs shake most obviously when they are at rest. The symptoms disappear when sleeping or consciously moving the limbs.

Tremors have a greater impact on the extremities. Symptoms are usually only present in one hand or one foot at first,

Chapter 2. What is Parkinson's disease？

but later spread to both hands and feet. The tremors of Parkinson's disease are often accompanied by hand movements of "robbing pills", that is, the patient's index finger will involuntarily move closer to the thumb. The two fingers circle each other, just like a pharmacist making pills.

Hypokinesia, another symptom of Parkinson's disease. The patient's movements become slower and affect the entire process from movement initiation to execution.

The patient is unable to perform consecutive movements or perform different movements simultaneously. Bradykinesia is a type of Hypokinesia. Bradykinesia means slowness of movement and speed (or progressive hesitations / halts) as movements are continued. This is a common symptom in the early stages of Parkinson's disease. Patients will initially have difficulty performing fine motor activities of daily living (Such as writing, sewing, or grooming). Clinical assessment is observed by asking the patient to perform actions similar to those described above. The impact of Bradykinesia varies with the type of movement and the patient's physical and mental state.

The degree of impact is affected by the patient's activity and emotional state. Some patients are so severe that they cannot walk, but some patients can still ride a bicycle. In general, people with Parkinson's disease improve in Bradykinesia after treatment.

The stiffness of the limbs is due to the patient's increased muscle tone and continuous muscle contraction, making it difficult to move the limbs. Rigidity caused by Parkinson's disease may be lead pipe rigidity (Fixed resistance) or cogwheel rigidity (Resistance is not fixed but regular). Cogwheel rigidity may be caused by tremors combined with increased muscle tone. The stiffness of the limbs in patients with early Parkinson's disease is often asymmetrical, and often occurs in the neck and shoulders. It then spreads to the craniofacial area and limbs, and finally spreads to the whole body as the disease progresses. Gradually, the patient loses his or her ability to move. I think that's what happens to me when I exercise, especially when riding a bicycle. My right foot often comes off the pedal and cannot pedal smoothly.

Chapter 2. What is Parkinson's disease？

Gait disturbance is one of the symptoms of late-stage Parkinson's disease. Patients may fall frequently due to poor sense of balance and may suffer fractures as a result. There is usually no gait disturbance in the early stages of the disease. Up to 40% of patients have fallen due to unstable gait during the course of the disease. The number of falls is related to the severity of the disease. During my illness, my walking was normal and I never had any falls.

Restless legs syndrome (RLS) is a common movement disorder that usually occurs at rest. It mainly refers to unbearable discomfort in the calf including severe pain and abnormal sensation in the calf. Restless legs syndrome (RLS) is common in patients with Parkinson's disease, with an incidence rate of 8% ～ 34%. It affects patient's sleep quality by interfering with sleep. It's pathogenesis may be related to dopaminergic system disorders, genetic mutations, abnormal iron metabolism, etc.

Other symptoms of movement disorders in Parkinson's disease include abnormalities in posture, speech, and swallowing. Patients may develop a Parkinsonian gait (or festinating gait, from Latin festinare [to hurry]) (Accelerating the pace and bending forward when walking) to avoid falling. They may also have difficulty speaking, have a masked face (Poker face), or micrographia. Patients may develop various movement problems. (This section is referenced and transcribed from the Internet search : Wikipedia / Parkinson's Disease / Motor Symptoms)

| Chapter 2.What is Parkinson's disease？ |

Parkinson's disease may cause mental and neurological disorders 03

A small number of patients with Parkinson's disease may develop mild to severe neuropsychiatric disorders, including confusion with speech, cognition, mood, behavior, and thinking.

Cognitive confusion may occur in the middle and late stages of the disease. The incidence rate increases with the duration of the disease. A more common cognitive deficit problem in people with Parkinson's disease is weak executive functioning. It will affect patient's planning, cognitive flexibility, abstract thinking, rule understanding, appropriate behavior, working memory, concentration, etc. Other symptoms of cognitive confusion include problems with concentration, inaccurate perception and estimation of time, and slow cognitive processing. The patient's memory will be affected. It is particularly difficult for the patient to recall previously learned information ; however, symptoms can be improved if clues are provided to assist the patient's recall. Loss of spatial awareness is another possible symptom. The test will ask the patient to recognize facial expressions and the direction of the lines to determine if the patient has this disorder.

People with Parkinson's disease have a risk of developing dementia that is approximately 2 ∼ 6 times that of the general population. The incidence rate increases over time. Dementia reduces the quality of life of patients and caregivers. It increases mortality. There is a greater chance of needing to be admitted to a nursing home.

People with Parkinson's disease who do not have cognitive impairment are more likely to have behavioral and mood disorders than the general population. These patients usually do not have dementia. The most common mood disorders are depression, apathy, and anxiety. However, people with Parkin-

Chapter 2. What is Parkinson's disease？

son's disease often present with symptoms such as dementia, reduced facial expression, hypokinesia, apathy, and dyskinesia, which makes diagnosing mood disorders more complicated. I recalled that during the course of my illness, I was often impatient with complex matters, would put off things, and was unwilling to face them. (This section is mainly referenced and transcribed from the Internet search：Wikipedia / Parkinson's disease / Neuropsychiatric Disorders)

Parkinson's disease and sleep disorders

Sleep disturbance is also a possible Parkinson's disease symptom. Medications used to treat it may worsen the problem. Patients will experience drowsiness, rapid eye movement interruption, insomnia, etc. Wikipedia describes a review report showing that 13.0% of patients with Parkinson's disease have sleep disorders.

Excessive daytime sleepiness (ESD) refers to sudden sleep without reasons during the daytime when the patient is awake. At present, the pathogenesis of ESD is not yet clear. It may be related to dysfunction of the ascending reticular system. According to research reports, about 50% of patients with Parkinson's disease are affected by ESD. It is more common in men and more common in people with depression. In some cases, ESD has a greater impact on patient's daily lives than the motor symptoms of Parkinson's disease.

Rapid eye movement sleep behavior disorder (RBD) is an abnormal sleep behavior related to rapid eye movement sleep (REM). This is a sleep pattern characterized by association with dreams. RBD patients are often accompanied by fear and violence during sleep. At the same time, they may have rapid muscle twitches and flailing limbs during the REM period.

My Parkinson's symptoms are relatively unrelated to my sleep problems. I rarely take naps at work, but I sleep well at night and rarely have nightmares. What interrupts sleep is mainly the contraction of the muscles of the right upper arm and the muscles of the right foot that want to stretch.

Majority of patients with Parkinson's disease have unknown etiology. Only a small percentage of patients can be attributed to genetic factors. Experts generally agree that Parkinson's disease is not caused by a single factor, but by a com-

| Emerging from the Shadows of Parkinson's Disease |

bination of factors, including environmental factors, age factors, genetic factors, etc. Other risk factors may also be related to Parkinson's disease, but causality has not yet been proven.

(This section is mainly referenced and transcribed from Internet searches : Wikipedia / Parkinson's Disease / Sleep Disorders)

Note 1."Understanding the Diagnosis and Treatment of Parkinson's Disease" by Dr.Pei-Haw Chen, Senior Attending Neurologist of the Geriatrics Team at MacKay Memorial Hospital---Mackay Hospital News-Issue 367, June 2020.
Note 2.Reprinted from the online article "Parkinson's Disease Just Started 6 Precursors, Symptom Detection, Treatment, and Life Expectancy in One Look".

Chapter 3
The brain—
The center for the onset of Parkinson's disease

Cause of Parkinson's disease

Common Parkinson's disease symptoms such as tremors, stiffness, slow movements, balance disorders, stiff facial expressions without a smile, and symptoms of depression are all related to the basal ganglia of the brain, which is the brain signal transmission center. After all, brain damage originates from free radicals. Free radicals can affect the mitochondria, which are where cells produce energy. After the so-called cellular power plants are interfered with by free radicals, the amount of energy they produce deteriorates and they tend to degenerate.

There is a place in the brain called the substantia nigra (A neural nucleus in the midbrain). There is a part in the sub-

| Chapter 3.The brain—The center for the onset of Parkinson's disease. |

stantia nigra called the pars compacta that secretes dopamine. This place is easily damaged by Lewy bodies. After being persecuted, it cannot secrete dopamine. If there is no way to secrete dopamine, it will directly affect our basal ganglia and obstruct its functions. Many of the executive functions of the brain have to go through the basal ganglia. It's like the role of a chairman and a general manager. The Chairman's vision has to be evaluated and implemented by the General Manager. It is similar to the role of turning on a red light or a green light. When there is enough dopamine, the green light is turned on. In short, it is the direct path, and the other indirect path is the character who applies the brake to the red light. Patients who lack dopamine cannot give the green light. If they want to take the first step to walk, they will pause for a long time and delay it. They will be slower when taking the first step. After taking the first step, they will start to keep walking. Not only Movement, thinking, and cognitive functions will also become slower, because the brain's thoughts go through the basal ganglia. (**Note 1**)

Most of the major symptoms of Parkinson's disease are caused by the degeneration of dopamine neurons in the substantia nigra pars compacta. The pathways that connect the basal ganglia to the outside world can be roughly categorized into five pathways depending on their projection locations: the motor, oculomotor, association cortex, limbic system, and orbital frontal cortex pathways. Because Parkinson's disease affects the transmission of messages upstream of the basal ganglia, all of the aforementioned circuits may be affected, causing Parkinson's disease patients to experience impairments in movement, attention, and learning. (This section is mainly referenced and transcribed from the Internet search: Wikipedia / Parkinson's disease / Pathophysiology)

1980, the prototype of the theory of motor circuits and the correlation between this circuit and Parkinson's disease were proposed, which had a great impact on the scientific community at that time. Although it was later discovered that the model could not explain some phenomena, some corrections were made. In this model, the basal ganglia are responsible for reg-

Chapter 3.The brain—The center for the onset of Parkinson's disease.

ulating the motor system to avoid activation at inappropriate times. When the brain determines that an action is to be performed, the basal ganglia will reduce inhibitory signals so that the action can be executed smoothly. Dopamine can inhibit inhibitory messages from the basal ganglia. Therefore, when the dopamine concentration is high, it can promote the smooth occurrence of movement instructions. When the dopamine concentration is low, the movement instructions will be inhibited by the basal ganglia. Patients with Parkinson's disease have lower central nervous system dopamine concentrations, resulting in reduced motor function. Based on this theory, drugs that increase dopamine concentration are often used for drug treatment. However, this result often leads to activation of the motor system at inappropriate times, resulting in involuntary movements of the body. (This section is mainly referenced and transcribed from the Internet search：Wikipedia / Parkinson's disease / Pathophysiology)

　　Pathologically speaking, patients with Parkinson's disease have degeneration of "substantia nigra nerve cells in the midbrain" and are unable to secrete the neurotransmitter "dopamine". Due to the lack of dopamine, they are unable to effectively communicate instructions from the brain.

| Chapter 3.The brain—The center for the onset of Parkinson's disease. |

Diagnosis of Parkinson's disease

Many celebrities have suffered from Parkinson's disease, such as Pope Paul II, Pastor Graham, former U.S. Attorney General Leonardo, Grammy Award-winning star Linda Ronstadt, world boxing champion Ali, Hollywood star Michael J. Fox, Davis Feeney who won the bronze medal in the Olympic Games, Robin Williams, Deng Xiaoping, Hitler, Taiwanese musician Li Taixiang, actress Fang Cen, singer Zhan Yawen, protest celebrity Ke Cihai, etc.

Parkinson's disease is a progressive disease that gradually affects the patient's nervous system and various parts of the nervous system. Parkinson's disease is more common in middle-aged and older people, but there are also cases of the dis-

| Emerging from the Shadows of Parkinson's Disease |

ease in young adults.

Actually, there are signs of Parkinson's disease. If it is discovered and treated early, the outcome is usually better. Taiwan Movement Disorder Society provides a simple "Parkinson's Disease Self-Detection Form" for people to self-test at home. If 3 of the following 10 conditions occur, it may be an early sign of Parkinson's disease. It is recommended to see a neurologist.

(1) Have your hands ever trembled when you were resting and relaxing?

(2) Is one arm bent and not swinging when walking?

(3) When standing or walking, does your body bend forward?

(4) The walking posture is messy and uneven, as if it is knotted or one foot is trailing behind?

(5) Writing becomes slower and the font size becomes smaller?

(6) Small steps and frequent falls?

(7) Do you often feel lazy and have no motivation to do

| Chapter 3.The brain—The center for the onset of Parkinson's disease. |

anything ?

(8) Do you often have pain in the back of your neck or shoulders ?

(9) Deliberately avoiding friends or family members with whom you don't get along ?

(10) Is there a change in tone ? Has the tone become more monotonous, whispery, or raspy ?

Symptoms of Parkinson's disease vary from person to person. The rate of progression of each person is also very different. Symptoms of Parkinson's disease include:

(1) Hand trembling and limb trembling: In addition to limb trembling, patients may also rub their fingers.

(2) Muscle stiffness: All muscles of the patient's body may become stiff, making it difficult for the patient to move.

(3) Slowness of movement: The patient's movements become slow. Actions that were once simple now take more time and effort to complete. Walking pace is reduced, sometimes even walking with small steps or shuffling legs.

(4) Worsened sense of balance: Muscle stiffness and

tremors lead to a poor sense of balance for the patient, increasing the risk of falling and injury.

(5) Speech changes: changes in speaking voice, slurred speech, or hesitation before speaking.

(6) Difficulty doing fine movements: Some fine movements will be affected, such as cooking, writing or playing musical instruments.

Parkinson's disease can be divided into 5 stages according to the severity of the patient's movement disorder. The differences between different stages are introduced below.

Stage 1: The patient has symptoms on one limb, but it does not affect his or her daily life.

Stage 2: The patient has symptoms on both limbs but can still maintain balance.

Stage 3: The patient has difficulty maintaining a stable posture and is prone to falling.

Stage 4: The patient can barely stand and begins to need the care of others in daily life.

Stage 5 (final stage): The patient needs to be bedrid-

| Chapter 3.The brain—The center for the onset of Parkinson's disease. |

den or use a wheelchair for a long time, and needs professional care in daily life. (**Note 2**)

Although Parkinson's disease is a common disease, it is difficult to diagnose in the very early stages of the disease or in older patients. Doctors usually need to conduct a detailed disease history and neurological examination before making a diagnosis.

Some diseases have symptoms similar to those of Parkinson's disease, including slowness, stiffness or trembling when walking, including stroke, hydrocephalus, brain tumors, dementia, side effects of antipsychotic drugs, viral encephalitis, brain trauma, and hypothyroidism, vitamin B12 deficiency, etc., which must be differentially diagnosed with Parkinson's disease. (**Note 3**)

There is sufficient clinical evidence to point out that if you frequently fall, have symptoms that progress rapidly, or do not respond to anti-Parkinson drugs, you are more likely to have Parkinson-like syndrome rather than Parkinson's disease. Therefore, doctors must arrange relevant blood tests and brain imaging examinations, such as computed tomography (CT), magnetic resonance imaging (MRI) or brain dopamine neuron tomography (TRODAT), etc., to make relevant differential diagnoses. (**Note 3**)

Drug treatment of Parkinson's disease

Parkinson's disease is a degenerative disease. Symptoms such as stiffness, tremors, slowed movements, and difficulty in balancing indicate that the brain has degenerated to a certain extent and requires treatment. Early treatment can help delay the progression of the disease. If hand tremors are found, in addition to Parkinson's disease, it may also be due to neuropathy, brain tumors or thyroid problems. Once the diagnosis of Parkinson's disease is confirmed, treatment should be initiated aggressively.

Dopamine in the brain not only regulates movement, but also regulates mood, sleep, etc. Therefore, in addition to the more familiar motor symptoms, Parkinson's disease may also present many non-motor symptoms, such as depression, constipation, pain, sleep disorders, changes in sense of smell, etc. Some non-motor symptoms will appear earlier than motor symptoms. It is also important to seek medical attention if found to be relevant.

Parkinson's disease is a chronic disease. As the disease progresses, medications need to be adjusted in a timely manner. Therefore, seeking medical treatment nearby is one of the keys to ensuring regular return visits and discussions with the doctor. After receiving treatment for Parkinson's disease, patients and family members can record medication diaries, including medication time, motor symptoms, non-motor symptoms, sleep status, possible side effects, etc. During the follow-up visit, the doctor can evaluate whether medication needs to be adjusted based on the medication diary. (**Note 4**)

Before, Parkinson's disease was untreatable. Early symptoms were usually treated with levodopa. When the effect of levodopa diminished, dopamine agonists were used. As the disease progresses, neurons will continue to be lost, so the

| Chapter 3.The brain—The center for the onset of Parkinson's disease. |

dose of the drug must be increased accordingly. However, when the dose is first increased, involuntary dyskinesias will occur as a side effect. (This section is referenced and transcribed from the Internet search : Wikipedia / Parkinson's / Treatment)

Dosage fluctuations in medication can have a serious impact on patient's lives. When the patient first takes the drug, the dose in the body is higher, so the patient's symptoms are milder, which is called the "on" state. On the contrary, after the drug effect decreases, the patient's motor symptoms will appear again. At this time, it's called the "off" state. Excessively high doses of levodopa can cause dyskinesias in patients. Increasing the drug dose without limit is not a way to control the drug concentration in the "on state". Therefore, other methods must be used to prolong the retention time of drugs in the body, including the combined use of dopamine receptor agonists and MAO-B receptor inhibitors. In the past, doctors would temporarily discontinue levodopa to reduce motor symptoms, but this approach may lead to fatal side effects of Parkinson's hyperthermia syndrome, so it is no longer used. Currently, some manufacturers have developed intravenous and intestinal sustained-release technology to release levodopa stably and slowly. Studies have shown that sustained-release formulations are more effective in reducing dyskinesia than traditional formulations. Most patients must take levodopa for life, but patients taking larger doses may experience motor side effects of the product in the future. (This section is referenced and transcribed from the Internet search: Wikipedia / Parkinson's / Treatment)

Current treatments for Parkinson's disease include medication, surgery, focused ultrasound therapy, physical therapy, speech therapy, etc. Among them, drug treatment mainly restores the activity of dopamine so that the basal ganglia can maintain normal operation. There are currently six categories of drugs for treatment, including Levodopa, Dopamine agonists (DA), monoamine oxidase inhibitors, N-methyl-D-aspartate receptor (NMDA), Catechol-0-methyl transferase (COMT) inhibitors and anti-cholinesterase, among which

| Chapter 3.The brain—The center for the onset of Parkinson's disease. |

levodopa is currently the most effective and oldest drug. (**Note 3**)

Clinicians consider the patient's symptoms and use appropriate drug combinations to achieve the so-called "honeymoon period" effect in the early stage. Some patients can even reach a stage where no symptoms are apparent.

Levodopa is the main treatment drug for Parkinson's disease and has been developed and widely used for nearly 60 years. Levodopa will be metabolized into dopamine by dopamine decarboxylase in the body, causing side effects such as nausea and vomiting in the gastrointestinal tract, and side effects such as stiffness in joint tissues. In the end, less than 10% of the levodopa reaches the brain for therapeutic purposes. In order to increase the concentration of levodopa reaching the brain, Roche Pharmaceuticals obtained the patent for benserazide, and Merck Pharmaceuticals obtained the patent for carbidopa. Both inhibit the activity of dopamine decarboxylase in peripheral tissues and are mixed with levodopa to form oral dosage forms (trade names: Madopar tablets and Sinemet tablets), thereby increasing brain concentrations of levodopa while reducing Parkinson's disease pill burden (polypharmacy).

Entacapone is a COMT inhibitor. Its main function is to inhibit catechol-o-methyl transferase. This enzyme metabolizes levodopa in the body and prevents it from reaching the brain. Stavelo launched in the United States in 2003, further blending entacapone with levodopamine and a slow-release capsule carbidopa, into an oral dosage form to further minimize the pill burden in Parkinson's disease. Its main clinical trial, First Step (2005 ∼ 2007), is a double-blind randomized clinical trial conducted in multiple countries and centers (including the European Union and the United States). It has been shown to improve symptoms better than the mixed oral dosage form of levodopa and carbidopa.

Although long-term inhibition of dopamine decarboxylase has not been associated with serious adverse effects and remains the mainstay of treatment, drugs that inhibit catechol-0-methyltransferase are not so lucky. Tolcapone, a drug

Chapter 3.The brain—The center for the onset of Parkinson's disease.

that inhibits catechol-0-methyltransferase, has been withdrawn from the market because it may cause liver toxicity. Entacapone may also increase the liver index by more than twice in patients with liver dysfunction or alcohol abuse.

Inhibiting certain enzymes throughout the body to achieve the design of specific drugs to specific target organs can easily lead to unnecessary systemic side effects. It's like going from home to a certain place and not considering taking a car because you're afraid of being bitten by a dog on the way, but instead catching all the stray dogs and locking them up. But if stray dogs can chase away thieves, then if all stray dogs are locked up, there will be more thieves. Therefore, recent drug development has been moving towards the concept of drug carriers. Loading therapeutic drugs into specific carriers is like taking a car to the destination. In order to avoid being attacked by stray dogs, systems such as invisibility or bulletproofing can also be installed.

In order to reduce the pill burden of Parkinson's disease, drugs that are absorbed through the skin are also being developed. When drugs are delivered into the body through the skin, the stratum corneum is the biggest obstacle. The traditional method is to destroy or soften the stratum corneum. For example, chili paste improves drug delivery by destroying the stratum corneum. Recently, the concept of drug carriers has been gradually introduced. Nanosized carriers allow a specific drug to remain in a specific cortex for a sustained slow output, even up to tens of days.

Transdermal dopaminergic patches currently on the market are the transdermal patch Neupro ® marketed in the United States. Duodopa marketed in the EU is a kind of combination drugs of carbidopa and levodopa, clinical trials show Duodopa absorbed slowly from the small intestine. The two can effectively reduce body stiffness caused by dyskinesia or sudden power outage (off phenomenon), improve on phenomenon and reduce on-off fluctuation. For information on the treatment of Parkinson's disease, please refer to the Parkinson's Disease Treatment Recommendations of the Taiwan Movement Disorder Society. (**Note 5**)

| Chapter 3.The brain—The center for the onset of Parkinson's disease. |

Pill burden isn't just a problem for people with Parkinson's disease. It's a problem for many chronic disease medications. Through the research and development of drug delivery systems, reducing the number of pills and reducing systemic side effects is not a dream. I believe that in the near future, a new era of comprehensive personalized drug treatment will come. Any chronic disease can be treated with continuous drug delivery by simply wearing a watch and inserting a personalized disease card, without having to suffer the side effects of too many pills. (**Note 6**)

Deep brain stimulation surgery—DBS

This surgery inserts a neurostimulator into the brain, which then stimulates specific brain areas with electrical impulses. Deep brain stimulation surgery is generally recommended for patients whose motor symptoms fluctuate up and down. It is also suitable for patients with tremors whose symptoms are poorly controlled by medications or who cannot accept medications. (This section is referenced and transcribed from the Internet search: Wikipedia / Parkinson's Disease / Surgery)

The first line is to use drugs to treat essential tremor and resting tremor in Parkinson's disease. However, when some patients are not well controlled by drugs or cause serious side

| Chapter 3.The brain—The center for the onset of Parkinson's disease. |

effects, Deep Brain Stimulation Surgery will be considered to treat.

This surgery requires entering the operating room for Stereotactic Method and local anesthesia. Through craniotomy, a slender electrode wire is implanted into a specific nerve nucleus of the brain, such as the subthalamic nucleus, to electrically stimulate the operation of brain circuits and improve Motor function. At the same time, a battery must be buried under the skin of the chest to supply the current required by the electrodes in the brain. Therefore, the battery needs to be replaced in about 3 ∼ 4 years. Since it is necessary to open the brain to implant wires, electrodes, and install subcutaneous batteries, many patients are afraid, allergic to wires, or worried about the side effects of brain stimulation and are holding back. (NTU Newsletter Issue 1542 / Trembling No More ∼ NTU Hospital's press conference to learn about the "Shenbo Knife")

The first surgical treatment requires some out-of-pocket expenses, but National Health Insurance Administration (Taiwan) provides lifetime battery replacement benefits, with low surgical risks and few complications. However, it should be noted that deep brain stimulation surgery is not a surgery to cure the disease. Instead, the stimulation module needs to be adjusted over time and symptom needs, and combined with drugs to achieve further therapeutic effects. (Note 7)

In my data prior to receiving MRgFUS, deep brain stimulation was one of the options. Because this surgery was complex and not a one-and-done operation, I was deeply troubled and ultimately did not use it.

Note 1.Karl Li, DC, PT "Let's talk it together.":Agraland and Parkinson's disease.

Note 2. Reprinted from the online article "Parkinson's Disease Just Started 6 Precursors, Symptom Detection, Treatment, and Life Expectancy in One Look".

Note 3.("Understanding the Diagnosis and Treatment of Parkinson's Disease" by Dr. Pei-Haw Chen, Senior Attending Neurologist of the Geriatrics Team at MacKay Memorial Hospital---Mackay Hospital News-Issue 367, June 2020, page16~17).

Note 4. The above professional literature is referenced in Common Wealth Magazine Article-Care Online, Blog, January 11, 2024 "Treat mild hand tremors to avoid rapid deterioration~Monthly self-tests for early detection of Parkinson's disease".

Note 5.Parkinson's disease treatment recommendations from the Taiwan Movement Disorder Society ---Ac Ta Neuroloica Taiwanica, 2023 ;32:145 -184(Taiwan Journal of Neurology).

Note 6.Reprinted from "I don't want to be a medicine jar anymore! New developments in drug treatment of Parkinson's disease" written by Dr.Ming-Jun Tsai of China Medical University Hospital. China Medical News Issue 130.

Note 7.Transferred from National Taiwan University Hospital Parkinson's Disease Medical Center, "Shenbo Knife ～ MRgFUS !"

Chapter 4

Dawn appears—
Magnetic Resonance-guided Focused Ultrasound
(MRgFUS)

The origin and naming of MRgFUS

During a routine follow-up visit in August 2022, Dr.Chon-Haw Tsai told me that I could undergo MRgFUS（Shenbo Knife）treatment.

This is great news for me. I have been promoted from the observation list to the approved list, which is equivalent to seeing a light again from the rapidly worsening Parkinson's disease and being on the verge of death. Why does it carry so much weight in my perception？ According to the existing literature：

（1）It uses non-invasive focused ultrasound beam to perform thermal ablation in the brain at the lesion.

（2）General or semi-general anesthesia is not required.

Chapter 4. Dawn appears—Magnetic Resonance-guided Focused Ultrasound (MRgFUS)

(3) It can be improved for Parkinson's disease with mainly tremor. And according to the current reported literature, the efficacy remains unchanged four years after treatment. (**Note 1**)

What's more, there was no countermeasure that could reverse this disease before.

Although the doctor said that this is a new type of treatment and I don't know if there's a risk of relapse. I know that this large teaching medical institution has medical practices approved by Taiwan's health authorities. In addition, Parkinson's disease has never been irreversible for decades. My declining condition finally saw a chance of reversal, so I immediately agreed to participate in the treatment.

Taiwan is an aging society. The number of patients with essential tremor and Parkinson's disease is increasing year by year. Overall, the prevalence of essential tremor alone is about 4,000 ~ 40,000 per 1 million people ; among the elderly population over 60 years old, the prevalence is as high as 13,000 ~ 50,000 people. The "focused ultrasound" service

Emerging from the Shadows of Parkinson's Disease

initially provided by Taiwan's four major hospitals is a non-invasive treatment that integrates the teams of neurology, neuroimaging, neurosurgery. It provides an alternative for patients with primary tremors and Parkinson's disease. The full name of this technology is Magnetic Resonance-guided Focused Ultrasound. The abbreviation is MRgFUS. The Chinese nickname is "Shenbo Knife".

I told concerned friends around me that I was about to undergo Shenbo Knife, and after the treatment I no longer trembled. They were confused after hearing this, because Parkinson's disease only gets worse and worse. They have never heard that it will get better. What's more, it is a common disease among the elderly！

Why is it called "Shenbo Knife" in Taiwan？ Chon-Haw Tsai, director of the Department of Neurology of China Medical University Hospital, specially named "Magnetic Resonance-guided Focused Ultrasound" as "Shenbo Knife" when this technique was submitted to the health authorities for review in 2018. He believed that the Chinese character「神」

Chapter 4. Dawn appears—Magnetic Resonance-guided Focused Ultrasound (MRgFUS)

is pronounced "shen", which has the meaning of God's power and blessing, as well as the meaning of the nervous system. The tremors were immediately eliminated after treatment, which is really "amazing", that Chinese pronounciation is also "shen". Chinese character 「波」 is pronounced "bo" means that the source of treatment is focused ultrasound. Chinese character 「刀」 is synonymous with "knife" means treatment. Wherever the Shenbo Knife comes, the disease will disappear and be cured！It's so concise and powerful！

The healing principle of MRgFUS

In Taiwan, four major hospitals including China Medical University Hospital and National Taiwan University Hospital launched ultrasound-focused services in August 2022, integrating professional teams of multi-specialty medical staff such as neurology, neuroimaging, neurosurgery, and radiology. It brings more advanced medical services to patients with essential tremor and Parkinson's disease. My vision is focused on focused ultrasound unilateral thalamic cauterization！！

2016, scientists used focused ultrasound to cauterize the thalamus nucleus on one side of the human brain and found that the tremor symptoms of essential tremor could be improved by nearly 50%. The effects were maintained four years

Chapter 4. Dawn appears—Magnetic Resonance-guided Focused Ultrasound (MRgFUS)

after treatment.

The principle of focused ultrasound is to use high-power ultrasound to heat tissues at specific depths in the body with the assistance of special positioning instruments. When used in the brain, it can cauterize nerve nuclei and block the neural circuits that cause tremors. During treatment, a special helmet is used to focus 1024 ultrasound beams, and combined with the stereopositioning of brain MRI images, it can accurately cauterize the nerve tissue a few millimeters (mm) deep in the brain in a non-invasive way. Magnetic resonance imaging system is like the "eye" of the "Shenbo Knife", allowing doctors to identify and target lesions with high precision before and during treatment. Through the guidance of magnetic resonance imaging, a personalized treatment plan is developed for the patient. Magnetic resonance imaging is used to monitor the temperature changes of the target lesion in real time during the operation to ensure that the energy is focused on the target lesion. Immediately, magnetic resonance imaging (MRI) is used to confirm the signal changes after treatment of the target lesion. In addition, this instrument can emit more than 1,000 beams of ultrasound, using ultrasound to accurately focus high energy on deep brain tissue to achieve therapeutic effects. During the treatment process, lower-energy ultrasound will first be used to focus on the treatment target of brain lesions, and then the patient's tremor response will be immediately assessed, including the relief of tremor and whether there are any unexpected reactions, such as weakness, numbness, and headache., dizziness, nausea, vomiting, etc. When the patient's tremor slows down and the confirmed lesion target is correct, the ultrasound energy is gradually increased so that it can accurately ablate the lesion. Patient's tremors can improve immediately after treatment.

The treatment process of Shenbo Knife does not require brain opening or general anesthesia, which greatly reduces the risk of infection and bleeding. This procedure uses magnetic resonance imaging and high-energy ultrasound, has no radiation, does not require a craniotomy, and does not require implants.

Chapter 4. Dawn appears—Magnetic Resonance-guided Focused Ultrasound (MRgFUS)

Common side effects accounted for 20% of the subjects, and the vast majority were transient dizziness, nausea, vomiting, weakness, numbness, headache, or abnormal gait. Generally, it will disappear within 1~3months of follow-up. According to 4-year follow-up literature reports, Shenbo Knife cautery improves essential tremor, and the effect is still improved by 60 ~ 70% in the fourth year, and there are no lasting side effects.

Clinical application: Health authorities in the United States and Taiwan approved focused ultrasound for the treatment of patients with essential tremor in 2016 and 2017. At present, this treatment has not been included in the health insurance benefits. Patients who receive the treatment need to pay for it themselves. The fees of each medical institution vary. The basic hospitalization course is three to four days. After admission, you will receive a pre-treatment examination and arrange focused ultrasound treatment. You can be discharged from the hospital the next day, and then return to the outpatient clinic for follow-up treatment.

Focused ultrasound is more widely indicated in Parkinson's disease. Food and Drug Administration's approval in 2018 that "focused ultrasound cauterizes unilateral basal ganglia can treat tremors with poor drug response in Parkinson's patients", in November 2021, the U.S. Food and Drug Administration has approved focused ultrasound to cauterize the globus pallidus to treat Parkinson's dyskinesia. Prior to these approvals, only two medical institutions had reported small clinical trials showing that focused ultrasound for unilateral pallidus cautery improved motor complications in patients with Parkinson's disease, including "off" state are reduced by about 30 ∼ 40%, and dyskinesias are improved by about 40 ∼ 50%. In addition, Insightec has launched an international clinical trial (PD006；international trial number：NCT03319485) since 2017 to study the efficacy of ultrasonic pallidum cauterization in Parkinson's disease. The locations of the subjects include the United States, the United Kingdom, Israel, Canada, Japan, South Korea, and Taiwan. Although the official trial results have not yet been published, according to

Chapter 4. Dawn appears—Magnetic Resonance-guided Focused Ultrasound (MRgFUS)

the internal analysis data provided by Insightec to the U.S. Food and Drug Administration, the trial results found that about 70% of the subjects had a therapeutic response to the globus pallidus cautery. After 12 months, there was an overall reduction of about 30 ∼ 40% in the number of off state and dyskinesia. Based on this exciting preliminary trial report, the U.S. Food and Drug Administration approved focused ultrasound unilateral pallid cautery for the treatment of moderate to severe Parkinson's disease in November 2021. This reinforces the importance of this technique in the clinical management of Parkinson's disease. It is expected that after the cross-team focused ultrasound treatment in major hospitals is launched, it can provide patients with essential tremor and Parkinson's disease with new treatments that do not require surgery.

As for whether each patient is suitable for performing this technique, it still needs to be evaluated by a movement disorder physician at the neurology department's outpatient clinic before making appropriate arrangements. (**Note 2**)

The term transcranial magnetic resonance guidance mentioned here refers to the MRI magnetic resonance imaging machine. Magnetic Rresonance Imaging (MRI) is different from X-ray examination or CT computer scanning. It does not cause radiation and it's effect on the human body is greatly reduced.

Magnetic Rresonance Imaging (MRI) can capture the tissues and structures of internal organs in the body from multiple angles, allowing doctors to see clear images of the patient's brain, bones, heart and other entire bodies.

MRI examinations take 20 to 60 minutes. They are painless and require no anesthesia. They do not involve ionizing radiation and there is no worry about absorbing radiation. This MRI is like a tunnel machine. The patient can lie down and slide into the tunnel for examination. Conditions that can be diagnosed with a brain MRI scan including:

Brain inflammation, masses, and structural problems can also diagnose, intracerebral hemorrhage, cerebral blood vessel aneurysms, stroke, traumatic brain injury, etc.

Magnetic Resonance Imaging (MRI) does not re-

Chapter 4. Dawn appears—Magnetic Resonance-guided Focused Ultrasound (MRgFUS)

quire intrusion into the human body. It can obtain arbitrary cross-sectional views of various structures and tissues of the human body, and it can also obtain numerous other physical parameter information. MRI examination has not been found to have any side effects on the human body for more than ten years in the world. It does not produce ionizing radiation and is not invasive to the human body. Therefore, no matter how many times it is used, it will not cause radiation damage to the human body like traditional inspection methods such as X-rays. It can scan in multiple directions, provide three-dimensional images, and has High contrast resolution and other advantages.

The latest MRI model (Signa MRI Infinity Excite) has faster imaging speed and higher image resolution. It provides faster, more detailed and clear high-quality images, so that there will be no hiding place for any disease. It can help clinicians to take good care of the public's health and achieve early diagnosis and preventive health care. (**Note 3**)

Magnetic resonance imaging system is like the "eye" of the "Shenbo Knife", allowing doctors to identify and target lesions with high precision before and during treatment. Through the guidance of magnetic resonance imaging, a personalized treatment plan is developed for the patient. Magnetic resonance imaging is used to monitor the temperature changes of the target lesion in real time during the operation to ensure that the energy is focused on the target lesion. Immediately, magnetic resonance imaging (MRI) is used to confirm the signal changes after treatment of the target lesion.

Cases of using MRgFUS to treat tremors

Shenbo Knife was first used to treat patients with essential tremor. In 2019, the 74-year-old Mr.C prepared for a major turning point in his life according to the scheduled process. In addition to his dear children, the people who accompanied him through the entire turning process included a complete medical team, including neurosurgeons, surgeons, neuroradiologists, researchers and nursing staff. Each medical staff had formulated a complete treatment evaluation plan before Mr.C was hospitalized to ensure that Mr.C could obtain satisfactory treatment results.

Mr.C is a patient who has suffered from essential tremor for more than 10 years. This neuro degenerative disease is not necessarily a fatal emergency, but the gradually severe tremor of his hands will cause great inconvenience in daily life. Small things that most people find easy, such as writing with a pen, raising a glass to drink water, shaking hands with others, etc., cannot be completed smoothly. As a result, many patients develop symptoms such as low self-esteem, social withdrawal, and even depression.

After many clinical studies, neuromedical experts have found that as long as a low-energy ultrasound beam is focused on the ventral intermediate nucleus of the thalamus on one side of the patient, the tremor of the patient's contralateral hand can be significantly improved.

The advantage of this treatment is that the patient does not need to bear the risk of surgery, remains awake during the entire treatment process, and does not require general or partial anesthesia. It is a suitable treatment method for most elderly people suffering from this disease. Because the clinical safety and effectiveness of this "Magnetic Resonance-guided Focused Ultrasound" (Referred to as Shenbo Knife in Tai-

Chapter 4. Dawn appears—Magnetic Resonance-guided Focused Ultrasound (MRgFUS)

wan) has been proven in many countries around the world, the U.S. Food and Drug Administration (FDA) announced in July 2016 MRgFUS was approved to treat essential tremor. Taiwan's Ministry of Health and Welfare also approved its use for domestic patients in November 2017. With the cooperation of many factors, Mr.C became the first patient to receive Shenbo Knife treatment at China Medical University Hospital.

During the treatment process, the medical team accurately calculated and controlled the energy of 1024 ultrasound probes to confirm the location of the ventral nucleus lesion in Mr.C's left thalamus. When the ultrasound energy given reached a certain level, Mr.C was surprised to find tremor symptoms

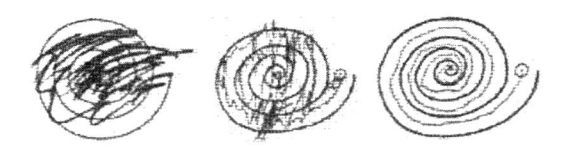

The picture above from left to right shows the spiral diagram drawn by Mr.C with a pen in his right hand before treatment, during treatment and after treatment.

in his right hand disappeared. After the treatment, he picked up the cup next to him and took a sip of water freely. He was moved and said that he could finally drink water from the cup with his own hand！He had been waiting for this moment for several years. (**Note 4**)

Chapter 4.Dawn appears—Magnetic Resonance-guided Focused Ultrasound (MRgFUS)

My MRgFUS treatment experience

04

At the early stage of my treatment for Parkinson's disease, I had already gone through a diagnostic evaluation prescribed by an outpatient physician, and the assistant staff of the neurology team evaluated the relevant actions. When the date for the Shenbo Knife treatment was scheduled, the Neurology Team Assistant again asked me to come in for a more in-depth evaluation. This is about two hours of muscle stretching, movement and thinking evaluation. It included installing sensing buttons on the muscles of the head, arms and feet to test the response of muscle surfaces to electrical currents. I was walking on a carpet with voltage to record the walking pressure of the two feet ; and video recording of various body movements, etc. In order to compare the differences between preoperative and postoperative improvements. Another very important step is MRI-the location of the lesion before treatment is determined by magnetic resonance imaging. (Transferred from National Taiwan University Hospital Parkinson's Disease Medical Center, "Shenbo Knife ~ MRgFUS！")

Pre-treatment positioning：The success of focused ultrasound cauterization greatly depends on the accuracy of the cautery position and the focus of the ultrasound energy. Therefore, before receiving treatment, patients must first undergo brain magnetic resonance imaging (MRI) to confirm information such as the nerve structure and blood vessel direction in the brain. They must also undergo skull computed tomography imaging to confirm skull density ratio, SDR) is suitable for such treatment. The actual method is to use a stereotaxic head frame externally fixed on the head to provide coordinate guidance, allowing doctors to locate a specific small area in the thalamus called the ventral intermediate nucleus of thalamaus (Vim). Since there is no natural boundary between

Chapter 4. Dawn appears—Magnetic Resonance-guided Focused Ultrasound (MRgFUS)

the nerve nucleus and other nerve nuclei in the thalamus in the Vim interface, the normal human brain structure norm will be used as the benchmark point for the test. Skull bone density: Those with skull bone density greater than 0.4 are more suitable for focused ultrasound treatment and require preoperative brain computed tomography for judgment. The MRI takes about 40 ～ 50 minutes. It only does the head and not other parts of the body. It does not require anesthesia or imaging agents. It feels very relaxed and comfortable. (Transferred from National Taiwan University Hospital Parkinson's Disease Medical Center, "Shenbo Knife ～ MRgFUS ! ")

Then there were written instructions for Shenbo Knife procedure. I was also informed in advance that the hair should be shaved. I was told to prepared with elastic socks and diapers for the hospitalization. Diapers are required because the treatment lasts up to four hours. It will be inconvenient if I have to get off the machine to pee midway. Wearing elastic stockings is to prevent some people from having blood clots caused by poor blood flow in their legs. I didn't pee in the diaper afterwards, but a deeper level of precaution was necessary.

Then I was admitted to the ward and prepared for the treatment of Shenbo Knife.

On the first day of hospitalization, a medical assistant will come to the ward to determine if any supplies are lacking. Director Chon-Haw Tsai came with six or seven doctors and interns to confirm that my symptoms such as drawing circles, trembling hands and feet, and verbal expressions were videotaped. And made sure I stopped taking Parkinson's and other drugs.

The first thing I did the next day was to shave my hair again, using a razor until it was so smooth that the roots of my hair could no longer be touched. After putting on socks and diapers, the doctor who operated the Shenbo Knife equipment put on a helmet made of alloy, which looked like a crown. Its function is to ensure that the position of the head will not deviate from the position where the Shenbo Knife is to be performed as the patient's shoulders and neck move. After all, this position is just a small point, and the brain is densely packed

Chapter 4. Dawn appears—Magnetic Resonance-guided Focused Ultrasound (MRgFUS)

with billions of thoughts and instructions, every point has its function that can not be deviated from.

In addition to putting on the helmet, it also need to tighten the screws on the helmet, which will cause a painful tingling on the skull. Therefore, the doctor will apply a small dose of anesthetic to the area of the scalp where the screws are to be tightened. This is the only painful part of the whole process.

So, I wore a helmet, took a wheelchair from the ward, and was pushed to a special room. The main thing inside was a huge machine, much like a larger MRI, and there was also a monitoring room. There were already about ten experts inside, wearing doctor's white robes, witnessing the entire process.

Everyone's getting busy. Some people check the monitoring equipment, and some people check the water, electricity, etc. of the machine. I wear a tight silicone cap inside my helmet, a bit like the little hats worn by Jewish men. Its function is to allow ice water to flow in the cap when the Shenbo Knife focuses the heat on the lesion to cool it down, so as to prevent the brain from being unable to withstand the high temperature and being damaged.

I lay down on the MRgFUS table and put earplugs in my ears. They worried that the sound waves would make me uncomfortable because I was going to undergo ultrasound. Then the technician put a button switch in my hand and said that if I felt very uncomfortable, just press the button and the members in control room would know. I don't have access to these thoughtful designs. In fact, the whole process is just lying down.

"Shenbo Knife" focused ultrasound is to use high-power ultrasound to heat tissues at specific depths in the body with the assistance of special positioning instruments. When used in the brain, it can cauterize nerve nuclei and block tremors. During the treatment, a special helmet is used to focus 1,024 ultrasound beams, and combined with the stereopositioning of brain magnetic resonance imaging, it can accurately cauterize the neural tissue a few millimeters deep in the brain in a non-invasive way. (**Note 5**)

As a patient, I didn't know how to operate the Shenbo

Chapter 4. Dawn appears—Magnetic Resonance-guided Focused Ultrasound (MRgFUS)

Knife beforehand. During the first round of about ten minutes, I heard the sound of water flowing above my head, and my ears were filled with the high-pitched knocking of "Di ∼∼ Di ∼ ∼" sound, and then exit the tunnel entrance of the machine. A bunch of people came to me from the monitoring room. I felt that my hands were still shaking and my feet were shaking slightly.

These people were busy with their own business, some were checking my helmet, some were looking at the ice water system……I only heard Director Tsai told me in a very firm tone: "Now, we need to strengthen it a little more！"

"Di ∼∼ Di ∼∼", "Di ∼∼ Di ∼∼" The knocking sounds are more rapid and sharp. However, after the second, third, and fourth rounds, my right hand was still shaking. At this time, the shoulder and neck reflect soreness, pain, and numbness, which is very uncomfortable. It turns out that Parkinson's disease causes shoulder and neck pain, but I can only feel it when I lie down.

The whole process of Shenbo Knife involves the patient

first receive low-energy focused ultrasound on the machine to stimulate the preset Vim area, and then slowly increase it to high energy. During the step-by-step advancement process, each stimulation will cause a brief heating of a small area of the brain. Through a temperature imaging device, medical staff can sense the heating effect of ultrasound energy on brain tissue from a distance. During the step-by-step positioning test and energy improvement process, medical staff will also enter the monitoring room to assess the patient's tremor symptoms. When it is determined that the test area can achieve the greatest symptom improvement, the highest energy cauterization is performed to raise the temperature of the brain tissue to the therapeutic temperature (Approximately 56 degrees Celsius), thereby achieving permanent cauterization. (**Note 6**)

In the fifth round, I felt that the sound waves were stronger and the pressure on the top of my head was stronger. My shoulders were a little sore and uncomfortable. I had been lying down for a long time and wanted to change my sleeping position, but it was better not to move around. I had to endure

Chapter 4.Dawn appears—Magnetic Resonance-guided Focused Ultrasound (MRgFUS)

it. About fifteen minutes later, the machine stopped running and I exited the tunnel again. Surprise! My hands are no longer shaking, and my feet are no longer shaking! My whole body stopped shaking! I was so surprised that I felt the air seems to have frozen.

After getting off the machine, I immediately stretched out my right hand, stretched out five fingers, looked at the front and back, and then stretched them out to show Director Tsai. I shouted: "I won't shake anymore!" In order to avoid dizziness, I was eager to take off my helmet at this moment, because the helmet now became a burden that was hanging tightly on my head. Under the arrangement of the assistant, I was afraid that I would be dizzy and unsteady, so I sat in the wheelchair again. Under the guidance of Director Tsai, I followed him to do some hand and foot exercises of Parkinson's disease. And then he asked me how I felt now? I replied, "I'm not shaking now. It seems that the treatment was successful and deserves applause!" All medical staff, technicians, and interns at the scene also applauded involuntarily. The scene suddenly felt like a celebration !

I was Immediately removed the helmet and silicone head cap. The treatment was successful ! I felt as if a thousand kilograms of burden had been lifted.

The Department of Imaging Medicine of National Taiwan University Hospital has drawn up the "Shenbo Knife treatment process". The content is easy to understand. I excerpt it here for the reference of people from all walks of life.

"Shenbo Knife" treatment process:

(1) Patient preparation: Before treatment, computed tomography and magnetic resonance imaging scans are performed to assess suitability for treatment. On the day of treatment, the hair was shaved preoperatively and local anesthesia was applied to fix the stereotaxic frame. The patient lies supine on the treatment bed, with his head placed in the "Shenbo Knife" helmet, and cooling water is circulated around the scalp to cool down.

(2) Treatment plan: Develop a treatment plan and identify treatment targets by combining preoperative and intra-

Chapter 4. Dawn appears—Magnetic Resonance-guided Focused Ultrasound (MRgFUS)

operative magnetic resonance imaging.

(3) Target verification: During treatment, lower-energy ultrasound is first used to focus on the treatment target, and then the energy is gradually increased to conduct an immediate assessment of the patient's response.

(4) Treatment: High-energy ultrasound is used to accurately focus energy on the target point, and magnetic resonance imaging is used to continuously monitor temperature changes in the target area in real time. Gradually increase the target temperature to about 60 degrees to cause thermal ablation of the target tissue.

(5) Assessment (after treatment): Use spiral drawing or other testing methods to evaluate improvement in tremor. After the last ultrasound treatment, the magnetic resonance imaging image is scanned to confirm the ablation area.

Average treatment time is 2 ～ 3 hours.

| Emerging from the Shadows of Parkinson's Disease |

Note 1.See the article "Shiver no more" in issue 1542 of the NTU newsletter, and search for the article "Transcranial Magnetic Vibration-guided Focused Ultrasound" in the web site of the China Medical University Hospital.
Note 2.Transferred from National Taiwan University Hospital Parkinson's Disease Medical Center, "Shenbo Knife ～ MRgFUS ！"
Note 3."Introduction to Magnetic Resonance-guided Focused Ultrasound（Shenbo Knife）" at China Medical University Hospital.
Note 4.Written by Dr.Ming-Kuei Lu, Dr.Jui-Cheng Chen, and Director Chon-Haw Tsai of the Department of Neurology, China Medical University Hospital, "Gathering the magical power of thousands of ultrasound beams. Shenbo Knife successfully treats essential tremor", April 15, 2020---China Medical News No. 192.
Note 5."Trembling is No More" Press Conference of National Taiwan University Hospital（Shenbo Knife）---National Taiwan University News Issue 1542.
Note 6.Transferred from National Taiwan University Hospital Parkinson's Disease Medical Center, "Shenbo Knife ～ MRgFUS ！"

Chapter 5
After MRgFUS treatment

How you feel immediately after surgery

After leaving Shenbo Knife machine, I returned to the ward and took a nap for more than two hours. The medical staff said in advance that after the treatment, the brain will be weak due to the energy-consuming effects of burning, so more sleep will be needed. Actually, I woke up from my nap with cramps in my legs. I haven't had foot cramps in sleep or while hiking for more than ten years. Now I have cramps in both legs, which I find very peculiar. Next, I walked from the ward to the tea room to get water to drink. It was about 20 meters away. As I walked, I felt that my right foot could not keep up with the pace and would drag. The toes of my right foot would deviate from the normal position.

Chapter 5. After MRgFUS treatment

In the aforementioned chapter "The healing principles of Shenbo Knife", I quoted from the Parkinson's Disease Medical Center of National Taiwan University Hospital: "Common side effects (Referring to Shenbo Knife) account for about 20% of the subjects, and the vast majority are short-term dizziness, nausea, weakness, numbness, headache or gait abnormalities, generally disappear within 1 ～ 3 months of postoperative follow-up." The Phase II clinical study, BEST-FUS Trial 2, published in the July 2021 issue of Movement-Disorder, a journal of neurology, noted that bilateral thalamic focused ultrasound cauterization can still achieve curative effect in patients with essential tremor; however, after three months of follow-up, 7 out of 10 patients experienced minor side effects, such as: slurred speech, difficulty swallowing, and unsteady gait, etc.

On my third day in the hospital, that is, the day after the treatment, when Director Tsai brought four doctors to me for inspection, I also stated the above-mentioned abnormalities I noticed to the doctors. In the next two weeks, my cumulative postoperative abnormalities included:

(1) Abnormal gait, only on the right side, and my right foot could not keep up with the stride of my left foot.

(2) The muscles of the right upper arm are still tightened inward, and the finger strength of the right hand is not as good as that of the left hand.

(3) In terms of oral expression, the vocabulary used is not clear and comprehensive, the words are simplified, and the tone is low, which makes the listener feel strange.

(4) Inability to walk long distances. Walking about 800 meters at a time is the limit, and then I have to sit down and rest.

Fortunately, these conditions improve naturally after three to five months. The most obvious thing is that my speech has reached a state of satisfaction within 3 months. For example, singing, I'm supposed to be good at it! At the beginning, I had some difficulty in articulating words, but after five months I was able to sing a song perfectly. As for nausea, vomiting, numbness, and headaches, they have never happened to me.

Chapter 5. After MRgFUS treatment

And I can walk longer and longer.

No more medication after treatment and no reason to take medication！

Director Tsai also arranged for regular follow-up visits, and the evaluation team members will conduct post-operative evaluation for me. They also conducted more than a dozen tests in the past two hours, and also arranged for an MRI to determine the signal changes in the focal target of the lesion after treatment. During a follow-up visit half a year after the treatment, I squatted up and down with my heels and toes on the ground faster and faster. I responded to Director Tsai：

"I feel better & better！" When I saw Director Tsai smile, I couldn't help but laugh too.

Although the symptoms of discomfort are naturally subsided, my right foot is still a little unable to keep up with the stride length of my left foot. The muscle tightening in my right arm still affects my vision and my movements look strange. By chance, I met a Chinese medicine practitioner who is well versed in acupuncture and "Acupotomology". It mainly uses shallow needles to prick the fascia of the muscles to loosen the fascia of the muscles. When I traveled to Thailand, I received the "hammer tendon" pose for massage, use a mallet to tap the tendons. As a result, both of them have a positive effect on my hands and steps. The muscle tightening in my upper arms has disappeared, and the inability of my right foot to follow my left foot has disappeared. The difference between my hands and feet is only in carrying the suitcase. There is a slight difference when loading weight, but generally no difference is visible.

Summarize the seven major advantages of Shenbo Knife treatment:

(1) No radiation.

(2) No need for craniotomy.

(3) No implants.

(4) No anesthesia is required and the patient is awake during the entire treatment process.

(5) Accurate thermal fusion + controllable temperature.

(6) The risk of postoperative infection and bleeding is

extremely low.

(7) Quickly return to normal life after treatment.

Therefore, it is an extremely safe and immediately effective one-time treatment. During the three days of treatment, I was not accompanied by my family. After I was discharged from the hospital, I took a bus to eat egg cakes and drink soybean milk. In short, I was relaxed and at ease.

Current situation one and a half years after MRgFUS treatment

About a year after the Shenbo Knife treatment, I signed up to participate in a walking event with thousands of people. I walked on a large road in the mountainous area. There were slight ups and downs, but not much. The total distance was 6 kilometers. I walked to the end. I felt exhausted before the point, so about 6 kilometers was my bottom line. Unexpectedly, one and a half years later, because my feet exert stronger force and my steps up and down the stairs become more natural, I can now walk 18,000 steps a day including going up and down the stairs. I used to be afraid of climbing, but now I can walk on the trails in Dakeng Mountain District in Taichung City. The uphill slope is about 30 degrees, which is not a problem. The downhill is even easier, and

Chapter 5. After MRgFUS treatment

I no longer feel exhausted.

My pronunciation when singing was a bit inaccurate three months after treatment. Now, even if I encounter fast-paced songs, I can sing smoothly. It's just that when dancing, when encountering fast-paced steps, sometimes the natural reaction is to combine three steps into two steps, resulting in a disordered step！I think the nerves in my legs still need to be exercised over time, and they should get better and better.

I once tried jogging, such as walking through an intersection. When the light signal was about to end, I would jog and speed up, but I couldn't continue running. The main problem is that when running fast, there is a slight discrepancy in the coordination of the steps of the right foot, just as when dancing, the pace of the fast tempo can not be kept up.

When I hold a spoon or fork in my right hand and put food into my mouth, it used to tilt and cause the food to fall in advance. Now I can eat very stably without falling.

The expression on my face has completely changed. My face, which used to be very serious and silent, has become smiling and soft, which is recognized by everyone who has seen me before and after.

I am optimistic that once the dopamine secretion in the brain reaches a normal state, the instruction given by the brain to learn will stimulate the neural circuit and once again enhance the motivation to try. By repeatedly outputting the learned information and practicing, my movements will become better and better.

The Hebbian theory in neurology mentions that "continuous and repeated stimulation of presynaptic neurons to postsynaptic neurons can lead to an increase in synaptic transmission efficiency." In other words, "repeated stimulation of neurons increases the synaptic strength between neurons." Therefore, continuous movement can improve imperfect movements, including running and dancing.

Therefore, the treatment mode of Shenbo Knife is not just a way to "cut off" nerves, but to remove roadblocks and then "reorganize" the degenerated tissues, allowing dopamine nerve cells to secrete normal concentrations of dopamine again, thereby eliminating the symptoms of Parkinson's disease. Through repeated stimulation of neurons, the normal state of body movements is restored.

Conclusion

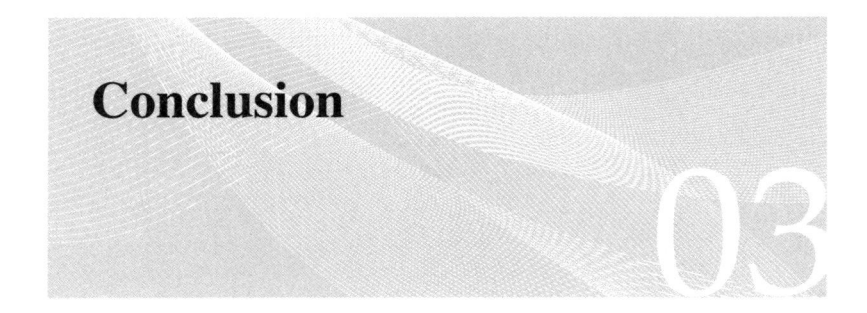

In the past, it was believed that after Parkinson's disease was diagnosed, its condition would not stop or be controlled by taking drugs. The treatment for Parkinson's disease symptoms was usually levodopa or other related drugs, which may become worse over time. It will cause side effects, such as patients having abnormal limb twisting (dyskinesia), so it is very important to accurately stabilize the concentration of the drug in the blood.

In addition to medication, there is a treatment modality called deep brain stimulation (DBS). The surgical procedure is to place slender electrode leads on the patient's brain, and implant the generator near the sterno-collar bone (Similar to

Chapter 5. After MRgFUS treatment

the installation location of the heart rhythm regulator) and connect it to the leads. It uses electric current to regulate incorrect messages in the brain, thereby improving the patient's symptoms. But deep brain stimulation surgery still cannot completely treat Parkinson's disease.

Shenbo Knife treatment on me can be said to have opened a window of opportunity for the medical profession in the treatment of Parkinson's disease.

Shenbo Knife treatment, the tremors will stop immediately. Although there may be symptoms such as slurred speech, unsteady walking, and nausea, these will gradually fade over time and even improve as the movements become stronger.

For Shenbo Knife to improve or stop the downward spiral, to improve my physical fitness, to improve my inconvenience of life's movements, to regain self-esteem in life, to remove the dependence on drugs, and to remove the shadow of death, all have happened to me with immediate and significant results.

The day after my treatment, a group of intern doctors

came to see my condition. I told them briefly : "You are in the right department. Neurology plus Shenbo Knife can help thousands of patients and their families to be free from pain ! "

During my return visits to the Department of Neurology at China Medical University Hospital, I unconsciously held Dr. Chon-Haw Tsai's hand several times and said "Thank you" to him, expressing my infinite respect and gratitude.

Currently, the magnetic resonance guided focused ultrasound therapy system has been approved for clinical treatment in many countries, such as the United States, Europe, Israel, Canada, South Korea, Japan, China, Thailand and Australia.

Shenbo Knife is suitable for non-invasive treatment of small lesions. It has also been developed and conducted in many studies at home and abroad, such as controlling neuropathic pain, delivering drugs to specific organs or tumors, and assisting in opening the blood-brain barrier to aid in the efficacy of chemotherapy for tumors, thrombolysis, and psychiatric-related disorders such as depressionn, etc. Shenbo Knife

| Chapter 5.After MRgFUS treatment |

has a wide range of applications and has the advantages of minimal trauma and precision, so its role will become increasingly important. (Note 1)

At present, more than 6 million people worldwide suffer from Parkinson's disease, and only a few people have received medical information from MRgFUS. Of course, whether MRgFUS is needed or other treatment methods are suitable depends on the doctor's evaluation and judge. However, it is a true fact that Shenbo Knife completely cured my Parkinson's disease. I am making my lucky medical experience public and hope that Shenbo Knife can bless those in need and improve everyone's quality of life. Have a safe, healthy, happy and beautiful second half of your life.

Note 1."Trembling is No More" Press Conference of National Taiwan University Hospital (Shenbo Knife) ---National Taiwan University News Issue 1542.

觀成長

走出巴金森病幽谷：神波刀讓我重拾美好人生
(中英對照)

作　　者—張正駿
視覺設計—徐思文
主　　編—林憶純
行銷企劃—蔡雨庭

總 編 輯—梁芳春
董 事 長—趙政岷
出 版 者—時報文化出版企業股份有限公司
　　　　　108019 台北市和平西路三段 240 號
　　　　　發行專線—（02）2306-6842
　　　　　讀者服務專線—0800-231-705、（02）2304-7103
　　　　　讀者服務傳真—（02）2304-6858
　　　　　郵撥—19344724 時報文化出版公司
　　　　　信箱—10899 台北華江橋郵局第 99 號信箱
時報悅讀網— www.readingtimes.com.tw
電子郵箱— yoho@readingtimes.com.tw
法律顧問—理律法律事務所　陳長文律師、李念祖律師
印　　刷—勁達印刷有限公司
初版一刷— 2025 年 2 月 21 日
定　　價—新台幣 350 元
版權所有 翻印必究
（缺頁或破損的書，請寄回更換）

時報文化出版公司成立於 1975 年，並於 1999 年股票上櫃公開發行，於 2008 年脫離中時集團非屬旺中，以「尊重智慧與創意的文化事業」為信念。

走出巴金森病幽谷：神波刀讓我重拾美好人生
（中英對照）/ 張正駿作. -- 初版. -- 臺北市
: 時報文化出版企業股份有限公司, 2025.02
　　216 面 ; 14.8*21 公分 --（觀成長）
中英對照
　　ISBN 978-626-419-048-0（平裝）

　　1.CST: 巴金森氏症　2.CST: 超音波療法
　　415.9336　　　　　　　　　　113018093

ISBN　978-626-419-048-0
Printed in Taiwan.